The Zero Trimester

The Zero Trimester

PRE-PREGNANCY CARE AND THE
POLITICS OF REPRODUCTIVE RISK

Miranda R. Waggoner

UNIVERSITY OF CALIFORNIA PRESS

University of California Press, one of the most distinguished university presses in the United States, enriches lives around the world by advancing scholarship in the humanities, social sciences, and natural sciences. Its activities are supported by the UC Press Foundation and by philanthropic contributions from individuals and institutions. For more information, visit www.ucpress.edu.

University of California Press
Oakland, California

Library of Congress Cataloging-in-Publication Data

Names: Waggoner, Miranda R., author.
Title: The zero trimester : pre-pregnancy care and the politics of
    reproductive risk / Miranda R. Waggoner.
Description: Oakland, California : University of California Press, [2017] |
    Includes bibliographical references and index. | Identifiers:
    LCCN 2017010811 (print) | LCCN 2017013124 (ebook) |
    ISBN 9780520963115 (ebook) | ISBN 9780520288065 (cloth : alk.
    paper) | ISBN 9780520288072 (pbk. : alk. paper)
Subjects: LCSH: Reproductive health—21st century. | Women—Health
    and hygiene—21st century. | Pregnancy—Complications—21st century.
    | Women's health services—Political aspects—21st century. | Public
    health. | Health risk assessment.
Classification: LCC RG133 (ebook) | LCC RG133 .W338 2017 (print) |
    DDC 618.2—dc23
LC record available at https://lccn.loc.gov/2017010811

Manufactured in the United States of America

25 24 23 22 21 20 19 18 17
10 9 8 7 6 5 4 3 2 1

Dedicated to

Dr. Lorraine V. Klerman (1929–2010), cherished mentor, influential scholar, and stalwart advocate for maternal and child health

Contents

Acknowledgments

The idea for this book originated years ago, while I was hiking in New Hampshire with one of my graduate-school mentors, Lorraine V. Klerman. I had just read the CDC's guidelines for pre-conception care, and Lorraine had recently served on the CDC's expert select panel on pre-conception care. I had many questions about the emergence of this seemingly new idea for improving birth outcomes and how it might interface with cultural assumptions about gender, risk, and responsibility. A renowned public-health scholar, Lorraine was always very patient with and intrigued by my sociological interest in the relationship between medical knowledge and social order, and she helped me turn a project idea into a reality.

Along with her unwavering intellectual support and expansive knowledge on my subject, Lorraine's connections to leaders in maternal and child health were key to the development of my project. Soon after our hike, in her usual collegial spirit, Lorraine invited Kay Johnson and me to her home in Waltham, Massachusetts, to discuss the history and potential implications of a pre-conception care framework in public health. Kay was lead author on the CDC's pre-conception care guidelines, and her expertise on the subject ran deep. Kay's encouragement was absolutely essential to the trajectory of my work, and she expedited my research in numerous ways, including supporting my attendance at the third National Summit on Preconception Health and Health Care. Additionally, Dr. Hani Atrash pleasantly welcomed me to CDC offices in Atlanta to pursue my research.

I am truly grateful to all the experts who took time out of their busy schedules to talk with me about pre-conception care. I learned so much from them, and I admire their dedication to healthy mothers and children. I realize that all of the professionals with whom I spoke will not agree with some of my arguments in this book, but I hope that my work will engender future dialogue about that which we indubitably share: a commitment to maternal and child health. I am in awe of the everyday work they all do in this realm and am thankful to be part of the conversation.

I am intellectually indebted to my mentors at Brandeis who were central in the development of this project. For years now, Peter Conrad has nurtured my thinking on this topic and many others, and his general equanimity kept me grounded during the uncharted journey of writing a dissertation and then a book. His knack for big conceptual thinking molded my own analytic mind in important ways. Karen V. Hansen facilitated my intellectual interest in the intersection of medicine and motherhood, and I thank her for being a model scholar and person. Sara Shostak helped me tremendously as I navigated key questions in the sociology of medicine and science. After Lorraine passed away, I was quite distressed, and Susan Parish graciously and competently stepped in as a policy expert during the latter stages of my dissertation research and provided essential assistance and support.

It is no secret that Elizabeth Mitchell Armstrong's work has profoundly influenced my own. After crucially helping me formulate key arguments during my dissertation work, Betsy invited me to Princeton to study as a postdoctoral fellow. To say that this was a fortunate opportunity would be a massive understatement. During my time at Princeton, I was able to work with and talk with Betsy on a weekly basis, and I learned a terrific amount about how to navigate research projects, academia, and life. Betsy is a wide-ranging intellectual, a consummate mentor, and a kind friend. Thank you, Betsy, for making all this possible.

Susan Markens and Norah MacKendrick read countless drafts of chapters and were enduringly understanding and encouraging, uplifting me with their optimism, smart commentary, and good cheer. They were able to reveal clarity where I saw only blurred ideas, and they were quick to insert a thought-provoking comment where I most needed it. I am not sure the final manuscript would have come to fruition without them. For their camaraderie and friendship, I am immensely and continuously grateful. Rene Almeling and Kristin Barker offered extremely helpful insights in the early stages of this book project and read the penultimate manuscript in full. Their thoughtful and careful observations and suggestions vastly improved my work. Of course, any failings in this book are my own; but, for any of the book's successes, I share them with my mentors, and Susan, Norah, Rene, and Kristin.

Additionally, a number of colleagues—including Elizabeth Chiarello, Michaela DeSoucey, Bridget Gurtler, Joanna Kempner, Erika Milam, Jan Thomas, Ashley Rondini, Rebecca Flemming, Keith Wailoo, and anonymous reviewers at *Signs* and *Journal of Health Politics, Policy and Law*—read earlier versions of chapter sections and conference papers and offered very useful commentary. Over the last few years, my thinking on this topic has been enriched by conversations with Elizabeth A. Armstrong, Angela Creager, Cynthia Daniels, Kathleen Ferraro, Kathleen Gerson, Chris Gillespie, Larry Greil, Carole Joffe, Kelly Joyce, Martine Lappé, Emily Mann, Christine Morton, Lynn Paltrow, Jennifer Reich, Deana Rohlinger, Lindsay Stevens, and Shirley Tilghman.

A version of Chapter 6 previously was published as "Cultivating the Maternal Future: Public Health and the Prepregnant Self," in *Signs: Journal of Women in Culture and Society* 40(4) (2015): 939–62. Several paragraphs throughout the text were previously included in "Motherhood Preconceived: The Emergence of the Preconception Health and Health Care Initiative," published in *Journal of Health Politics, Policy and Law* 38 (2013): 345–71. Thanks to the University of Chicago Press and Duke University Press, respectively, for reprint permission.

While researching and writing this book, I benefited from generous institutional and financial support from Brandeis University, Princeton University, the University of Virginia, Florida State University, the National Science Foundation, the National Institutes of Health, the Andrew Mellon Foundation, and the Eastern Sociological Society. Alexandra Turner, Hena Wadhwa, and Harry Barbee provided helpful research assistance at various stages of this project, and Heidi Muir was a delight to work with during the interview transcription process. Judy Hanley, Cheryl Hansen, Kay Bennett, and Nancy Cannuli also provided critical help with technical and administrative concerns at different moments in this project's trajectory. Naomi Schneider, my editor at the University of California Press, buoyed me with her thoughtful patience and consistent support for this project. Renée Donovan and Nicholle Robertson were considerably helpful during the production process. And Gabriela Whitefield's heartwarming and steady friendship during this time has been more vital than she knows.

I have been fortunate to spend time in multiple academic institutions over the past decade and a half, and throughout my time in each location, I received crucial support from colleagues and friends that sustained me in significant ways. When I was an undergraduate at the University of Texas, Christine Williams inspired me to pursue a career in sociology, and I also thank Marc Musick, Sharmila Rudrappa, and Gideon Sjoberg for their indispensable support during my time in Austin. During my years at Brandeis, Ashley Rondini, Ken Sun, Vanessa Muñoz, Tom Mackie, Meredith Bergey, Amanda Gengler, Sonja Jacob, Dana Zarhin, Giusi Chiri, Erin Rehel, Maia Hurley, and Nelli Garton were all brilliant friends to have as I began to traverse the world of academia. Special thanks are in order for Liz Chiarello who made my time at Princeton infinitely more humorous and intellectually stimulating than I could have imagined. Also at Princeton, I treasured my chats with Fah Vasunilashorn, and James Trussell provided steadfast support along the way, for which I remain very grateful. Michaela DeSoucey and Sarah Thébaud have been consistently lovely sources of friendship and wisdom—on topics sociological and maternal—since the day we met in New Jersey. From the University of Virginia, I thank Jeff Olick, Charlotte Patterson, Katya Makarova, and Corinne Field for their support. I feel privileged to have written the final version of this manuscript while among my wonderful and engaging colleagues at Florida State University.

My parents, John and Linda Waggoner, have provided support I cannot possibly recount, as it has been abundant and every day. They championed my educational path and intellectual pursuits from the very beginning, regularly took care of my young son so that I could work, consistently served as a sounding board for life and career questions, helpfully read chapters and listened to my arguments, and provided much emotional and gastronomical sustenance during the years of this project. Needless to say, I am deeply grateful. I also want to thank my grandparents, David and Leta Andrews, for being so inspirational and loving, and my late grandparents, Weldon and Adelle Waggoner, whom I miss dearly.

Finally, I end with a happy and wholehearted thanks to my husband, Sven Kranz, and our son, Anton—both came into my life during this work and brought love and joys unforeseeable and indescribable. Cliché, of course, because it's true: there are no words.

1 Someday, Now

PRECONCEIVING RISK AND MATERNAL
RESPONSIBILITY

Having a healthy pregnancy is no longer contingent on being pregnant in the first place. In February 2016, the federal Centers for Disease Control and Prevention (CDC) released a statement urging women of reproductive age to avoid alcohol if they were not using birth control, lest they harm a pregnancy that might or might not be present. The idea was vast: the CDC indicated that about 3 million American women were putting potential pregnancies at risk, but any woman between 15 and 44 years old was defined as "pre-pregnant," thus targeting, in effect, about 61 million American women.[1] This measure attracted considerable social commentary and ridicule,[2] but it hardly represented a new idea in public health. In 1981, Surgeon General Edward Brandt issued a warning that women "considering pregnancy" should refrain from alcoholic beverages.[3] Since 1992, Kentucky has required bars to post warnings that drinking alcohol *prior to conception* can cause birth defects[4] when, in fact, it cannot. The idea of pre-pregnancy health promotion surged after 2006, when the CDC released a report recommending improvement of the pre-conception health and health care of U.S. women of childbearing age.[5] Alcohol was just one of many pre-pregnancy risk factors listed in this report, and public health warnings issued since 2006 have not been limited to drinking.

In late 2012, for instance, Texas initiated a public-awareness campaign, called *Someday Starts Now,* for improving the health of the state's babies. In television spots, young women performed everyday activities—chatting with friends, exercising—accompanied by a looming bubble box filled not with dialogue, but rather with numbers indicating a long-in-the-future baby's due date, sometimes years away. This approach had the visual effect of dangling future motherhood above the women's heads. The campaign's associated website stated, "your health today is important—and even more important to the baby you might have someday."[6] The text further offered: "If there's a baby in your future, even if it's months or years from now, today matters. Take control. Stop smoking, eat right and exercise and do something about your stress."[7] After seeing this television spot, one blogger wrote, "Texas is Reminding Me I'm Just a Baby Vessel Again."[8]

The CDC and Texas campaigns represent but two illustrations of a growing tendency in medicine and public health to mark the beginning of healthy and responsible motherhood not at the birth or adoption of a child, not during pregnancy or at conception, but rather at an earlier point in time: pre-pregnancy. Similarly, in its recommendations for healthy pregnancy behavior, the March of Dimes—a national organization committed to improving birth outcomes in America—points directly to the three months prior to conception, claiming that a proper pregnancy today should actually last twelve months.[9]

These public health statements are jarring. Perhaps because of the invariant biological fact that a typical human pregnancy lasts about nine months, it is disconcerting to read that it instead should be thought of as a lengthier process. Given feminist progress over the past half century, the thought of women of reproductive age as primarily mothers-in-waiting seems problematic.[10] Also given that the focus on pregnancy health for more than a century has been on pregnancy behaviors, the thought of focusing on health behaviors *prior to* pregnancy is astounding. At the same time, these public-health assertions are somewhat expected. The sentiment that healthy babies stem from fit, responsible women echoes age-old societal preoccupations with women's bodies, behaviors, and reproductive outcomes. Anticipating and hedging future risk is reflective of our contemporary age of risk aversion and individualized responsibility for health. Concerns about the health of future generations have long manifested in cultural and political anxieties around family planning, fetal health, and women's roles in society.

Pre-pregnancy care is a framework that emerged as the new panacea for ensuring healthy pregnancies and healthy infants in the United States in the twenty-first century. It now is a dominant medical and cultural schema for reducing risks to healthy pregnancies, and it includes prescriptions for both health care and self-care. To have good pre-pregnancy health is to render pregnancy less risky, the thinking goes, and might improve the overall health of women, children, and society. What is emphasized, then, in contemporary health discourse is that for any woman of childbearing age, in the case of pregnancy health, someday *is* now.

Such messages are not coming only from health organizations. The notion of pre-pregnancy care has also entered the marketplace—touted as the fix for population health issues ranging from obesity to autism.[11] Women today can buy vitamins specially marketed for the pre-pregnancy period as well as advice books such as *Get Ready to Get Pregnant: Your Complete Prepregnancy Guide to Making a Smart and Healthy Baby.* Newspapers run headlines such as, "Start taking care of your baby before you get pregnant"[12] and "Don't focus on getting healthy while pregnant—do it before conceiving."[13] Even tabloids have expanded their surveillance rhetoric and routinely conjecture about whether celebrities are *potentially planning* a pregnancy through monitoring their day-to-day behaviors (e.g., "She was seen avoiding alcohol! She might be *thinking* about getting pregnant!").

What accounts for this current moment in which birth outcomes are defined in terms of a woman's whole adult life—well before she ever decided if and when to get pregnant and have a baby? What accounts for the contemporary reproductive landscape in which, as in the Texas health campaign, due dates are projected onto non-pregnant women and a healthy pregnancy is defined as lasting longer than nine months? How is it that now, in the twenty-first century, young women are essentially asked to act as responsible mothers before motherhood is their imminent reality?

This book confronts these questions by tracing the shifting boundaries of pregnancy health risk and maternal responsibility in America at the turn of the twenty-first century—by examining how and why the trend and task of perfecting pregnancies has extended at the front end of three trimesters. It proposes that this pre-pregnancy care model introduces a "zero trimester"—a concerted focus on the months or years prior to conception in which women are urged to prepare their bodies for a healthy pregnancy. The term "zero trimester" has not been previously used in academic, popular, or medical parlance; it is my own neologism that reflects growing sentiments among health professionals and others that individual women should adopt an attitude of anticipation when it comes to pregnancy health.[14] The zero trimester concept, then, refers to the period when a woman is not pregnant but when she is supposed to act *as if* she is pregnant.[15] The notion of the zero trimester is easily marketed as the three months prior to pregnancy, for example when organizations such as the March of Dimes claim that a pregnancy lasts twelve months.[16] This line of thinking, however, assumes that a woman will know exactly when she will conceive. Thus, the onus of pre-pregnancy maternal responsibility could be vast, without temporal bounds.[17] Some health professionals even point to a woman's lifetime of experiences as mattering to the health of a pregnancy. During my research for this book, one expert told me, without hyperbole, that "a woman is a mother from the time of her own conception." All of women's pre-reproductive years are in the zero trimester.

The idea of extended time for pregnancy has linguistic precedent, as the boundaries between discourses about fetuses and about newborns have become more fluid. The fetus has been represented and personified as childlike in popular and medical imaginations over the past several decades, parallel to both the work of pro-life activists as well as advances in medical technologies (such as sonograms) that render the contents of wombs visible.[18] Additionally, thanks to some popular infant-rearing and sleep books like *The Happiest Baby on the Block*, the concept of the "fourth trimester" has become part of many new parents' lexicons in recent years.[19] The "fourth trimester" idea denotes the difficult first three months after a child is born[20] and reflects the sentiment that these three months are essentially an extension of fetal development. As medical writer Susan Brink's book on the topic explains, "the fourth trimester has more in common with the nine months that came before than with the lifetime that follows."[21] For instance, the popularity of swaddling newborns—mimicking, in a way, life in the womb—is part of this extended-trimester framework.[22]

Thus, it is this cultural moment—one that has seen the rising importance of the fetus and expanding notions of trimesters—in which the zero

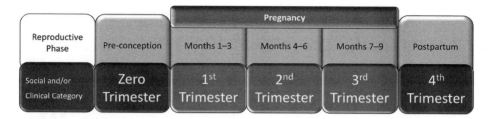

Figure 1. The twenty-first century pregnancy

trimester has materialized and flourished, changing, as it has, medical and social conversations about reproductive risk. Extending the fetal stage *prior to* as well as *beyond* pregnancy has become more typical within twenty-first century health-risk discourse. The zero trimester and fourth trimester are modern inventions, flanking the clinical period of pregnancy (*see* Figure 1).[23] In explaining the social and medical contours of how current health messages targeting women of reproductive age emerged, this book centers on the conceptualization of the pre-pregnancy period as a constructed trimester within a particular social, cultural, and political context of shifting ideas about risk and reproduction.

WHAT THE "ZERO TRIMESTER" INCLUDES

As mentioned above, contemporary pre-pregnancy care messages are informed by the U.S. Centers for Disease Control and Prevention's decision to begin promoting pre-pregnancy health and health care in the twenty-first century. In 2006, the CDC released a list of pre-conception health recommendations in the widely-circulated *Morbidity and Mortality Weekly Report* (MMWR), entitled "Recommendations to Improve Preconception Health and Health Care—United States."[24] This public health report was central to the emergence and trajectory of the pre-pregnancy care model. Following the release of the *MMWR*, the CDC convened a set of expert workgroups (clinical, public health, consumer, and policy) to filter recommendations and follow through with the report's goals. The result was numerous publications in the medical and public health literature about how to improve pre-pregnancy care among

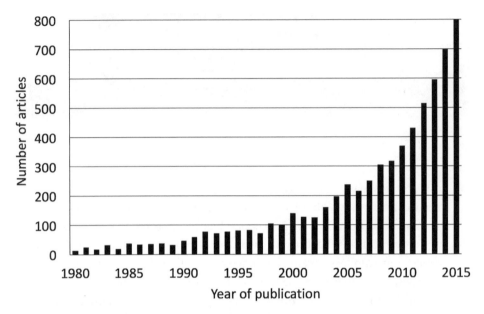

Figure 2. Number of publications on pre-pregnancy health or health care published in medical and health journals, 1980–2015

American women. More pre-pregnancy health promotion campaigns followed, and conversations within medicine and public health about pregnancy health quickly turned more squarely than ever before to the pre-pregnancy period (*see* Figure 2).[25]

With the manifest aims of reducing reproductive risk and improving birth outcomes—including infant mortality, maternal mortality, preterm birth and low birthweight—the basic idea of pre-pregnancy care is to advise and treat any negative health behaviors or conditions that might impact a reproductive-aged woman's future pregnancy. The *MMWR* outlined a concrete, though abstract, definition of pre-conception care as "a set of interventions that aim to identify and modify biomedical, behavioral, and social risks to a woman's health or pregnancy outcome through prevention and management."[26] According to the report, all providers who routinely see and treat women of reproductive age should be attuned to pre-pregnancy health and health care. They should be asking women— regardless of the nature of the clinical visit—what their reproductive plans might be and giving advice in accordance. The report also called for systematic changes in health care provision to offer additional coverage to pre-pregnant women. Women themselves are generally encouraged to partake in self-care, seek out testing (for genetic or hereditary predispositions and for sexually transmitted infections), take multivitamins (especially with folic acid), stop smoking cigarettes and drinking alcoholic beverages, and get conditions such as diabetes or obesity under control prior to conceiving. To an uncritical observer, these interventions might sound reasonable and desirable. That is, these recommendations carry a valence that is hard to argue with: Who would be against healthier mothers and babies? What became exasperating to some commentators is that the new model appeared to be a reawakening, of sorts, of the sentiment that women's bodies are only vessels for someone else—that women are mothers-in-waiting, and that it is the job of public health and medicine to control women's bodies for the sake of the greater good. In this way, observers pointed early on to how pre-pregnancy care might be perilous for women.[27]

Following the release of the CDC's 2006 report, media headlines engaged in both fear mongering and skepticism. The *New York Times* published an article entitled, "That Prenatal Visit May Be Months Too Late," and indicated that the guidelines applied to women of childbearing age even if they are not planning for pregnancy.[28] The *Washington Post*, in its article "Forever Pregnant," explained that "new federal guidelines ask all females capable of conceiving a baby to treat themselves—and to be treated by the health-care system—as pre-pregnant, regardless of whether they plan to get pregnant anytime soon" and that "so much damage can be done to a fetus" if recommendations are not heeded.[29] *Ms. Magazine* more directly pointed to the contentious nature of the new guidelines with the mocking title "Warning: You Could be Pre-Pregnant."[30] Popular outlets cautioned of potential fetal damage if women were not mindful of the new pre-pregnancy care guidelines, but also undermined the idea to a degree by noting that some might see the idea as outlandish.

It became clear following the CDC's report that different understandings of pre-pregnancy care were operating simultaneously. In one interpretation, public health officials were offering a forward-looking agenda to improve maternal and child health in the United States—a laudable goal to be sure. In another, critics began lambasting the idea of pre-pregnancy care as backward-looking and sexist. That such divergent viewpoints emerged shows that the idea of pre-pregnancy care struck a cultural and political nerve—something that I work to analyze and clarify throughout this book.

Indeed, the rise and meaning of pre-pregnancy care is much more complex and layered than critiques thus far have afforded. Intricacies abound in a close reading of pre-pregnancy care messages within medical and public-health discourse, revealing latent aims of the framework. For instance, proponents of this model situate it as an avenue for reproductive justice, a framework that includes improving women's reproductive opportunities and improving access to their reproductive needs. Yet, the contradictions are numerous and powerful. In one pre-pregnancy health webinar I tuned to in 2010, a renowned pre-pregnancy care expert expressed that if a woman chooses unprotected sex, she chooses a baby. This statement excludes various options women have once they conceive, and it also incorrectly assumes that unprotected sex is always a "choice" for women. When declarations like this one pepper discussions of pre-pregnancy care, it might be difficult for people to agree that it is a model for advancing reproductive autonomy. As argued in Chapter 4, the pre-pregnancy care approach does genuinely attempt to further reproductive justice, but of ongoing concern are unintended consequences that could stem from pursuing a model with a mindset that all pregnancies can be planned and that all women of reproductive age are potential mothers. Pre-pregnancy care might not simply be about improving birth outcomes, but also could be—as are most reproductive health agendas—wrapped up in the "longstanding societal ambivalence over the social roles of women."[31]

Furthermore, although some observers find pre-pregnancy care to focus on practical risk factors that might impact a woman's health and thus her future reproductive endeavors, such a seemingly straightforward risk-factor approach is accompanied by messaging that makes risk factors sound like *causes* of imperfect or adverse birth outcomes: if a woman engages in untoward behavior today, her future reproductive endeavors are at risk. The rhetoric of many pre-pregnancy health promotion materials mixes language of risk prevention with that of blame.[32] Take a CDC poster from 2009 that reads, "You just found out. You're pregnant! . . . It's too late to prevent some types of serious birth defects. . . . The time to prevent birth defects is *before* you know you're pregnant." This particular poster aimed to relay information about the potential of pre-pregnancy folic acid intake to reduce the risk of birth defects. Even though taking folic acid indeed reduces risk, *not taking* folic acid does not *cause* a birth defect. Further, the guilt-inducing, moralized message in this poster is somewhat inexplicable in that it seems to be a prevention message after the fact. Such messaging is presumably intended to make women aware of risk for their future pregnancies, to perhaps exploit what psychologists call "anticipated guilt."[33] In this way, it stokes the fire of critiques that pre-pregnancy messages place an undue burden on women of childbearing age. As I have found, the pre-pregnancy reproductive risk discourse of the twenty-first century evokes particular mechanisms and potential consequences for women that can be quite divisive. Indeed, some think pre-pregnancy care is irrational and others think it is essential. As revealed in the tenor of public-health messages that directly tie pre-pregnancy health behaviors to the risk of birth defects, it is also clear that this discourse is laced with sometimes-strident moral undertones, something to which I return in Chapter 5 and Chapter 6.

Although the notion of pre-pregnancy care was enlightening to some and maddening to others as it emerged on the national policy scene in the 2000s, the idea was not novel to many individuals working in fields of public health and medicine. There was momentum leading up to the CDC's report among those steeped in professional discussions about persistent adverse birth outcomes (*see* Figure 3). As early as 1980, a British physician wrote about the need for "pre-pregnancy clinics."[34] The Institute of Medicine's 1985 landmark study *Preventing Low Birthweight* was the first major medical publication to advocate changing the traditional point of obstetric care to the pre-pregnancy period,[35] addressing risk factors at the pre-pregnancy stage and stating that "numerous opportunities exist before pregnancy to reduce the incidence of low birthweight."[36] The 1989 Public Health Service publication *Caring for Our Future: The Content of Prenatal Care* adopted and expanded the concept of pre-conception care to include risk assessment, health promotion, and intervention follow ups, explaining that "the preconception visit may be the single most important health care visit" in terms of pregnancy and health outcomes.[37] *Healthy People 2000*, which targeted the nation's top health goals for the approaching decade, also highlighted pre-pregnancy health as a priority.

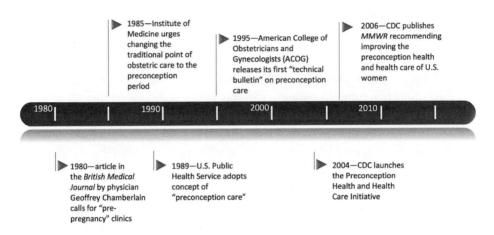

Figure 3. Key moments in the emergence of pre-pregnancy care, 1980–2006

As Chapter 2 discusses, physicians and public-health materials have emphasized the pre-pregnancy health of women for generations, albeit with different levels of intensity and specific concerns. Moreover, the idea of pre-pregnancy care is not new to those who might be proactive about pre-pregnancy genetic screening, such as those for whom genetic predispositions to certain diseases (e.g., Tay Sachs) are prevalent in their population group. Women and men who donate their genetic material to fertility clinics are often presented with a litany of health questions, and women and men who have faced infertility also might be acutely cognizant of pre-pregnancy care. For the vast majority of the population, however, health concerns around conception remain informal or nonexistent.

What is novel in the twenty-first century is the institutionalized nature of pre-pregnancy care as a model framework for reducing reproductive risk—an approach in which clinicians and public health officials now understand "proper" pregnancy care to include improving health behaviors, addressing risk factors, and pursuing treatments prior to pregnancy in a formalized way. As part of this framework, women are expected to care for their health prior to pregnancy. This includes planning their reproductive lives, improving lifestyle behavior, and seeking medical care. Moreover, clinicians are expected to assess women's health status prior to pregnancy and offer appropriate care interventions aimed at the woman as a pre-pregnant body. In practice today, this care framework serves as a main organizing principle for public-health campaigns, population health studies, and women's health care.

SITUATING THE ZERO TRIMESTER IN THE HISTORY OF PRENATAL CARE

It is impossible to understand the social creation of the "zero trimester" without understanding the historical rise and fall of the promise of prenatal care to improve U.S. birth outcomes. Prior to this century, most health professionals might have thought absurd the pre-pregnancy messages cited at the start of this chapter. The prevailing medical model for ensuring pregnancy health for almost one hundred years had been prenatal care— the idea being that if women engage in healthy behaviors and receive good clinical care *during* the nine months of pregnancy, then birth outcomes should be optimized and infant morbidity and mortality reduced.[38] The Children's Bureau first advocated clinical prenatal care in the early twentieth century,[39] but this concept did not take root as a universal expectation of pregnant women until the 1980s.[40] The '80s became known within the maternal and child health field as one of a "prenatal care revolution" because of the great increase in numbers of women seeking and accessing care.[41] Maternal and child health experts were hopeful that this surge in prenatal care utilization would reveal its "magic bullet" status, translating into vast improvements in population health. Quite surprisingly and contrary to the expectations of many, however, birth outcomes did not improve the more prenatal care American women sought and received. At the end of the twentieth century, infant health and survival in the United States ranked among the worst in the industrialized world and improvement in rates of adverse birth outcomes had stagnated.[42]

Such it was that a paradox had emerged—more and more women were accessing prenatal care services without parallel improvements in birth outcomes. When prenatal *care* seemed not to be doing enough, prenatal *education* was then pushed as the next big answer.[43] Sociologist Elizabeth Mitchell Armstrong writes that prenatal education, such as childbirth classes offered by hospitals, was "proposed as a solution to one of the most troubling social facts of contemporary America: despite the billions of dollars lavished on health care, despite ever-higher concentrations of medical technology, babies continue to die in this country at a much higher rate than elsewhere in the industrialized world."[44] Because many countries use infant and maternal mortality and morbidity rates as prox-ies for national health,[45] the United States did not distinguish itself as healthy or progressive in the 1980s. Experts began to question the evi-dence bolstering prenatal care. Maternal and child health scholar Lorraine V. Klerman wrote in 1990 that it was perhaps time to "question past ortho-doxies" and "loosen the link between prenatal care and infant mortality" because "public health experts know that the reduction of infant mortality requires much more than prenatal care."[46] In the interviews I conducted for this book, experts told me time and again that prenatal care basically does very little, if anything, to address the nation's most pressing maternal and child health problems.

Although prenatal care might be very effective at diagnosing and treat-ing problems that surface during a pregnancy, it does not prevent many of those issues from arising in the first place. It is especially ineffective at preventing the major causes of poor infant health outcomes: low birth-weight and preterm birth.[47] Moreover, health professionals are quick to note that almost half of U.S. pregnancies are unplanned, meaning that women often enter pregnancy without health care or healthy behaviors on their mind, and unintended pregnancies are often linked to a greater risk of an adverse birth outcome.[48] Many experts argue that U.S. women are just not healthy enough—and do not plan ahead well enough—and there-fore are putting the health of the next generation at risk. In this vein, and as Chapter 4 discusses in more detail, health experts began to question policies that only provide comprehensive health care to women when they are pregnant, rather than before and beyond motherhood. Thus, around the turn of this century, many maternal and child health professionals considered prenatal care—the perceived panacea for improving the popu-lation's birth outcomes—nothing more than a mere salve.[49] As one histo-rian has written, "prenatal care is no magic bullet and never will be."[50]

What was considered the best way forward? How do medical and pub-lic health experts tackle population health problems when the best idea to date has not worked? Near the turn of the twenty-first century, maternal and child health experts began contending that the answer to improving birth outcomes and to reducing infant mortality and maternal mortality was both prenatal care and *pre-conception care*,[51] or medical and health attention before pregnancy ever begins, in addition to care during pregnancy itself[52]—that is, to construct a zero trimester. If prenatal care seemed to be the answer for the twentieth century, then pre-pregnancy care would be the answer for the twenty-first.

In 2004, the Centers for Disease Control and Prevention launched the Preconception Health and Health Care Initiative, signaling a formal swing in policy focus toward improving women's health status through a focus on both individual women's self-care and improvement in health-care services for women of reproductive age prior to pregnancy. But how far prior? The answer was to move the temporality of pregnancy health risk and maternal responsibility to actions taken in the months—or sometimes even years—before pregnancy, thus situating essentially any body of reproductive age as posing risk to healthy reproduction.

This book examines this redefinition of reproductive risk; it is about a knowledge shift in the field of maternal and child health—about a search for a panacea in pregnancy care. It looks at the collective response to pressing population health and social problems when the clinical "fix" has failed, and it is about how a somewhat ambiguous idea of "pre-pregnancy care" came to "make sense" in medical and public-health discourse today.

DOES THE ZERO TRIMESTER MATTER? EVIDENCE AND AMBIGUITY

Of course, prenatal care did not become obsolete and instead has been bolstered time and again by social policy initiatives.[53] Prenatal care remains an "article of faith" in our culture,[54] and individuals, couples, doctors, health policy, and insurance companies continue to highly value it. To repeat, prenatal care does have individual-level benefits such as addressing and diagnosing problems that arise during a pregnancy, and the central argument of this book in no way posits that women's access to prenatal care services should be curtailed. What is germane here is that prenatal care does little in the way of *primary prevention*—a point that the medical experts I interviewed readily and repeatedly made. This means that prenatal care is reflective of our medical culture to treat rather than prevent.[55] It inscribes maternal responsibility as a "good" expectant mother seeking prenatal care throughout her pregnancy. Pre-pregnancy care, then, might seem an obvious next step for individuals and organizations immersed in the idea that seeking prenatal care marks responsible pregnancy behavior: if it is good, then the earlier the better. The added component of pre-pregnancy care was meant to complement, not supplant, the "old" prenatal model, and in so doing expand the sphere of medical and maternal responsibility for establishing healthy pregnancies.

Although the pre-pregnancy care model in some ways might be an empowering and smart way for women and physicians to approach family planning and reduce risk—and, indeed, the focus on pre-pregnancy care offers an important corrective to longstanding policies that have ignored the critical intersections between maternal health and reproductive health and that have in some ways impeded reproductive justice (a point explored at length in Chapter 4)—it in other ways might function as yet another attempt to control women and their behaviors, by placing their non-pregnant lives within new crosshairs of public scrutiny. To be sure, much of the criticism surrounding the pre-pregnancy care model has stemmed from the fact that pregnant women have long been construed as "public property" in America,[56] where, at an interactional level, strangers feel empowered to touch pregnant women's bellies and, at a structural level, the criminal justice system targets pregnant women for their behaviors. Surveillance of, and anxiety around, women's pregnant bodies remains typical. Imagine a visibly pregnant woman drinking at a bar in the United States; the social sanctioning that follows is perhaps inevitable. Then, imagine a non-pregnant woman drinking at a bar. Does anyone look at her and worry about her future fetus? Not likely. For a very long time, medicine, public health, and even the lay public have focused intently on policing a woman's behaviors when she is clearly pregnant. Few people—and few physicians—would think of telling a non-pregnant woman who drinks alcohol that she is possibly harming her chances of having a healthy baby someday. Yet this message is part of the CDC's 2016 public-health statements urging women of reproductive age to avoid alcohol. Even if the message might be well-intentioned in some respects, these types of directives run the risk of unintended consequences—namely of creating an atmosphere that escalates not only individual guilt among women but also social policing and public retribution against women who deviate from customary norms.

But is the hypothetical non-pregnant woman drinking at a bar actually endangering her future fetus? Do everyday choices and behaviors matter for future reproductive outcomes? It might make intuitive sense to be at one's healthiest before reproducing, but the evidence is ambiguous regarding whether specific pre-pregnancy behaviors will impact fetal health. With respect to alcohol, for example, the CDC's 2006 report stated that at "no time during pregnancy is [it] safe to drink alcohol, and harm can occur early, before a woman has realized that she is or might be pregnant" and that "alcohol-related birth defects can be prevented if women cease intake of alcohol before conception." Nowhere in this recommendation was the claim that *pre*-pregnancy drinking will affect the future health of the fetus or child. Rather, the predominant worry was that a woman will continue drinking without knowing she is pregnant. The public-health recommendation is to discontinue drinking *prior to* pregnancy so as not to continue drinking someday *during* pregnancy.

Although pre-pregnancy alcohol messages reveal how pre-pregnancy recommendations can be patently misleading and disingenuous, other examples allow us to better grasp the pre-pregnancy model's reasoning. There is good evidence to suggest that controlling certain chronic conditions prior to pregnancy improves individual chances for positive birth outcomes. For example, medical researchers have found that women with diabetes (both type 1 and type 2) are at increased risk of miscarriage and adverse birth outcomes, and that these risks can be mitigated through pre-pregnancy planning.[57] Another good example is HIV status, in which women who are HIV-positive could benefit from pre-pregnancy counseling about ways to prevent transmission to a future infant.[58] Moreover, public health officials and physicians are increasingly worried about widespread chronic conditions among women, such as obesity. Obese women have elevated risks for complications during pregnancy and childbirth,[59] and thus it might be very beneficial for such women to lose weight prior to pregnancy, both for their own general health and for their pregnancy health. At the same time, obesity has multiple causes and might not be easily remedied in a pre-pregnancy care visit. Other "epidemics" are troubling to health experts as well, such as the rising rates of opioid addiction among reproductive-aged women. Certainly, responsible health advice to a reproductively-capable woman who is addicted to opioids would be to avoid or delay pregnancy. Such advice, though, could be entirely unhelpful to the woman's broader life circumstances that situate her at risk for addiction, disease, or adverse birth outcomes.[60] Furthermore, while some pre-pregnancy risks are real, determining how individual risks—amid numerous social or environmental risks—become linked directly to birth outcomes might be telling for how and upon whom population health directives position responsibility. Is it possible to square the need to mitigate risk for particular individual women with the broad-based calls for all women of reproductive age to change their everyday behavior and act as if they are potentially pregnant?

As mentioned above, federal health reports have noted since the 1980s that a pre-pregnancy health-care visit might be of paramount importance to pregnancy outcomes. Since then, numerous organizations and scholars have touted pre-pregnancy care as the key intervention to improving maternal and child health in this country. But despite the faith expressed in pre-pregnancy care among many maternal and child health policy experts, there are significant gaps in clarity about the extent to which blanket recommendations to improve pre-pregnancy health and health care among all women of reproductive age will produce better birth outcomes in America.

First, temporal confusion abounds when it comes to discussions of pre-pregnancy care and the risk of adverse birth outcomes. The point of most pre-pregnancy behavioral interventions does not reflect evidence of clear connections between one's *pre-pregnancy* health behavior and identifiable fetal harm. Pre-pregnancy health discourse often actually is focused even more specifically on the *early pregnancy* period, *not* the pre-pregnancy period itself. With regard to smoking, for instance, the CDC has stated that of women who smoke, only 20% "successfully control tobacco dependence during pregnancy, [thus] cessation of smoking is recommended before pregnancy."[61] In other words, even for smoking—something generally considered to be bad for everyone—the principal concern is that women will not be able to stop smoking once they become pregnant and that women will continue smoking before they learn that they are pregnant, not that smoking at some point in one's life prior to getting pregnant equals increased risk for an adverse birth outcome.[62] Another example is folic acid consumption, which is covered in more detail in Chapter 2. Experts consider folic acid to be the best evidence for a pre-pregnancy intervention because of the effect it has on reducing the risk of neural tube defects such as spina bifida in developing fetuses. Folic acid is highly effective at reducing birth defects if it is consumed in *very early pregnancy*. Folic acid consumption thus might be a profound risk-reducing mechanism for women planning a pregnancy because they might become pregnant, but it does not reduce all risk of neural-tube defects and does not work through years-long consumption. Suggestions that folic acid should be consumed by all women of reproductive age throughout their reproductive years situates all such women as perpetually potentially pregnant. That is, with pre-pregnancy care messages and interventions, the focus no longer is on women at risk but on *all women of childbearing age*.[63]

Such widespread targeting stems from the fact that a key aim of pre-pregnancy interventions is to cover the periods of fertilization, implantation, and early pregnancy. In defense of the need for pre-pregnancy care, experts cite the first few weeks of embryonic development, which includes integral central nervous system and cardiac development, as a period when women are often unaware of their pregnancy and unintentionally forgo attentive health practices.[64] In as much as experts invoke scientific knowledge about the impacts of pre-pregnancy interventions, the chief hope is to target pregnancy intentions, a theme elaborated upon in Chapter 3. That is, the focus is on social behavior that foregrounds planning, and not on imminent medical risk. Pre-pregnancy care recommendations attempt to safeguard conception and early pregnancy because many pregnancies are unintended. Even women who intended to become pregnant, however, do not usually know the exact moment of conception. Thus, despite the temporal confusion of many pre-pregnancy health messages that falsely lead women to contemplate that every health behavior engaged in today might affect their fetus of tomorrow, zero tolerance now extends to the zero trimester.

Next, and more generally, we know very little about what actually causes most birth defects.[65] Studies point to a profound lack of etiological understanding of what makes a healthy—or unhealthy—pregnancy and birth, and medical experts often do not understand the root cause of most poor birth outcomes.[66] In fact, the two major causes of infant mortality—congenital anomalies and preterm birth—are not well understood by the medical community.[67] Moreover, in contrast to media-perpetrated stereotypes, most neonatal deaths occur among women in their twenties and early thirties who do seek medical care and who do not use illicit drugs.[68] In other words, the majority of adverse birth outcomes are to seemingly healthy women. Some measure of responsibility might lie with institutionalized medical practices, and not women's behavior. For example, analyses of the increase in preterm births find that high rates of labor induction, cesarean deliveries, and assisted reproductive technologies might be key drivers—factors that are not necessarily related to the pre-pregnancy health status of women but rather to the institutionalized culture of medical intervention in reproduction.[69]

Third, there are discrepancies in understandings about the health status of women of reproductive age. In recent population-based research, almost 89% of women of reproductive age reported good, very good, or excellent health, and about 75% of women of reproductive age had health coverage during the month before their most recent pregnancy.[70] At the same time, a quarter of women of reproductive age reported smoking cigarettes in the three months prior to pregnancy; about half reported drinking alcohol. Only about 30% reported taking a multivitamin or folic acid supplement.[71] These numbers lead experts to note that there is room for improvement in expanding knowledge about what constitutes good pre-pregnancy health. Even so, it is worth noting that we also do not know much about how pre-pregnancy health status has changed among women of reproductive age over the years; before the CDC's recommendations for improving pre-pregnancy care were published, few states monitored pre-conception health indicators specifically.[72] Data do exist, however, on general health behaviors and health risks of non-pregnant women over time. Such data suggest that some behaviors have improved since the CDC's recommendations, such as substantial reductions in smoking and drinking. Conversely, reports of binge drinking, obesity, or having diabetes, as well as self-reported health, all significantly worsened over the same time frame.[73]

Fourth, while the pre-pregnancy care framework attempts to address persistent and dramatic racial and ethnic health disparities in maternal and child health, it does so inadequately. Within the United States, such disparities are profound. Some women are more at risk of adverse birth outcomes, and some women—due to factors such as race, class, or geographic location—have poorer pre-pregnancy health than other women. The infant mortality rate for black women is double that of white women, a gap that has increased in recent years.[74] The maternal mortality rate for black women is more than three times that of white women and has also been on the rise.[75] While confronting the distressing reality of such inequalities in reproductive status and reproductive outcomes, pre-pregnancy health promotion materials have perhaps unwittingly reinscribed racialized notions of reproduction.

As Chapter 5 and Chapter 6 discuss in more detail, rather than addressing widespread social problems such as structural racism, poverty, or limited access to healthy food choices, our standard public health and medical agendas simply tell all women to practice the healthiest lifestyle possible to ensure healthy babies. Additionally, reproductive agendas in the United States are almost always racialized, built on contemporaneous ideas of "good reproduction" and engaging in what Rickie Solinger calls the process of "racializing the nation."[76] At issue is whether we are willing to focus our public-health interventions more squarely on reducing poverty- or race-based disparities for at-risk women rather than pursue policies that ask *all women* of reproductive age to change their behavior and plan their pregnancies without the supports they might need to do so.[77] Without systemic change, will only well-off women (or women seeking fertility services) be the ones to reap potential health rewards? We must ask who benefits from an expanded population health focus on pre-pregnancy health and health care.

Fifth, there is a deep disconnect in pre-pregnancy health materials between individual-level recommendations and social-level change in the landscape of maternal and child health. That is, beyond individual-level health risks and health behaviors there are, notably, vivid examples of environmental-level risks that harm non-pregnant individuals and that matter for their future birth outcomes. It is indisputable that birth outcomes have a lot to do with poverty and social conditions, including proximity to environmental contaminants before pregnancy. For instance, research reveals that long-term exposure to environmental toxins can damage genes.[78] In a 2015 exposé of the New York City nail salon industry, Sarah Maslin Nir of the *New York Times* revealed that nail technicians, by virtue of their prolonged exposure to chemicals, are at an increased risk of having a child with birth defects. Such cases of fetal or infant health risk have less to do with individual behaviors and lifestyle choices and more to do with widespread environmental exposures over which individuals have little control—calling into question the individualized tenor of many pre-pregnancy care messages. The pre-pregnancy care model today does incorporate messages for social change and awareness of the need for life-course approaches to holistic health, such as expanded health-care coverage for all women of reproductive age. As Chapter 5 and Chapter 6 show, however, overwhelming any system-level or environmental-level discourse are health-promotion messages directing every woman as to what she should do to improve her chances for healthy reproduction, including, in some instances, urging women to avoid particular activities or exposures. To keen observers, this advice could sound reminiscent of past "solutions" that aimed to bar women of reproductive age from toxic jobs—rather than eliminate the noxious exposure in the first place—to safeguard fetuses that are not yet conceived.[79] Pre-pregnancy risk factors epitomize a long-standing debate and tension in population health and public policy about how to navigate the relationship between individual-level risk and population-level prevention policies.[80]

Some of the debate about interactions between individual-level and environmental-level risk factors has been aided by the rise in social scientific concentration on cumulative life health[81] and epigenetics scholarship that links life-course outcomes to the time in the womb or even to the mother's lifetime experiences. The pre-pregnancy care model taps into the rise of these ideas. Scholars, however, have recently called-out such research for its inclination toward deterministic[82] and mother-blaming language. In a *Nature* essay in 2014, historian Sarah Richardson and colleagues situate contemporary epigenetics discourse in a long history of society blaming mothers for all kinds of children's health problems.[83] Although it has been argued that pre-pregnancy care is an extension of epigenetics research,[84] this book shows that the pre-pregnancy care literature predated the emergence of epigenetics as a popular scientific topic. Moreover, the experts I interviewed did not tend to couch the pre-pregnancy care model in an epigenetics paradigm. In fact, some saw epigenetics research as too simplistic, deterministic, and not necessarily concerned with the same things about which they were concerned. For example, the work of reducing unintended pregnancies—a key component of pre-pregnancy care—does not stem directly from epigenetics research. Rather, the pre-pregnancy care framework is gripped with broader ideas about—and politics surrounding—health care, family planning, motherhood, and reproduction.[85] So, while pre-pregnancy care might exist nicely in step with a postgenomic/epigenetic paradigm, it stands on its own historically and epistemologically.

Finally, men matter, but reproduction talk is almost always about *women*. It is a human creation that women's bodies are often solely tied to reproductive responsibility, yet such an arrangement appears as "common sense," as simply "the way things are." This sentiment is perhaps slowly changing. In her work a decade ago, political scientist Cynthia Daniels detailed at length how men's exposures to harmful chemicals, most pointedly with the example of Agent Orange in the Vietnam War, impacted their subsequent reproductive years, resulting in higher susceptibility for having children with spina bifida and other birth abnormalities.[86] Emerging science is showing more than ever that men's health status impacts the health of future fetuses. For example, men who smoke cigarettes damage their sperm's DNA, which might affect the health status of a future baby.[87]

Health behaviors might be particularly pertinent for men because, unlike eggs, new sperm is made every forty-two to seventy-six days, so "damaged" sperm can be replaced by newer "healthier" sperm within *three months* given a change in behavior or exposure[88]—in effect, the zero-trimester concept easily could be applied to men. To be sure, some pre-conception health materials mention men. For example, in Kentucky, the signs posted in restaurants and bars warning that drinking *before conception* can cause birth defects do so without express mention of women (this is unlike the Surgeon General's warning on alcohol that is usually explicitly addressed to women who are pregnant). This decision was made so as to include men—recognizing that men's pre-conception exposures might matter for reproductive health.[89] In Texas's *Someday Starts Now* campaign mentioned at the opening of this chapter and that featured television ads with images of women, web pages were devoted to both women's health and men's health and indicated that today's behaviors matter for future baby health "whether you are a man or a woman."

Yet, these mentions of men have been exceptions to the rule. As Rene Almeling and I have shown in previous work, men's contribution to reproductive health is still largely ignored or gestured to only nominally within the medical community broadly and within pre-conception health promotion materials specifically.[90] Overwhelmingly, the recommendations and rhetoric about pre-pregnancy care in promotional campaigns, and writ large, are still aimed at women—women who are not yet pregnant. Thus, while I do mention men and pre-pregnancy care at times, this book primarily focuses on how the zero trimester has been constructed for—and pitched to—women of reproductive age.

Given all of these considerations and such levels of uncertainty, one might wonder how pre-pregnancy care came to be seen as the panacea for improvement in birth outcomes. As Chapter 3 discusses, the pre-pregnancy care model has been bolstered and defined in the twenty-first century by obstetricians and health professionals who, rather than citing a clear body of scientific evidence, believe that this approach is "obviously" good for women and babies. If the evidence for pre-pregnancy health interventions is not particularly robust—or is, at the very least, quite scattered—then positioning the pre-pregnancy model as a foremost approach in reducing birth defects, infant mortality, or other adverse outcomes is questionable.

Is it ethical, or even reasonable, to tell women that the self-care and health-care behaviors they engage in today will influence the health of their future fetus, even when this might not entirely be the whole story—and especially if they have no power over the factors that might matter most?[91] The environmental and epigenetic examples provided above reveal that pre-conception harm might be at the environmental—rather than individual—level and might occur to men as well as to women. Nevertheless, the focus of the zero trimester is predominately on individual behavior change among women alone, not on men or social institutions. It is aimed at making and keeping a potential pregnancy in the forefront of women's minds at all times, often at the expense of focusing on systemic factors that might put women at lesser risk of unintended pregnancy or adverse birth outcomes in the first place.[92] Given these foci, it is imperative to analyze the tenor of the pre-pregnancy care approach to understand how population health strategies

are shaped—and also to critically assess how such a strategy hinges on medical science and on cultural assumptions and political sensibilities about
women, reproduction, and responsibility. Is this an instance of empowering
women or of making women feel guilty for birth outcomes that are not
solely—or even mostly—within their realm of control? Does pre-pregnancy
care place too great a burden on women of reproductive age?

To be clear, this book's aim is not to adjudicate the effectiveness of pre-
pregnancy care. As detailed above, some evidence suggests that it is incon-
sequential and misleading; some evidence suggests that it is profoundly
important. Proponents argue that this twenty-first century way of thinking about reproductive risk is the best and most effective path forward for
improving maternal and child health in America; critics argue that it is
pernicious and counterproductive and treats women unnecessarily like
baby vessels. This book, rather, focuses on why the magic-bullet solution
of "pre-pregnancy care" emerged when it did, particularly amid such variable interpretations of its message and effects, and what it tells us about
the contemporary politics of women's health, motherhood, and public
health prevention strategies. It scrutinizes the cultural and political logics
that have intersected with and informed the rise of a medical and public
health agenda in the early part of this century.

Sociologists of medicine and science have long observed that what has
become conventional medical and health wisdom is intricately tied up with
what is considered conventional social wisdom. That is, social, cultural,
and political currents shape and are shaped by scientific and medical
knowledge. I now turn to contextualizing the rise of the pre-pregnancy
care framework in such currents. Bolstering its emergence in the beginning of the twenty-first century were three overlapping trends: the perva-
siveness of risk discourse within surveillance medicine, the enduring
strength of motherhood ideology, and the ongoing fraught landscape of
reproductive politics and women's changing lives.

THE TEMPORAL (BIO)POLITICS OF HEALTH RISK

Part of understanding why and how the pre-pregnancy care idea emerged
when it did requires taking account of a broader trend related to risk. Risk

is today typically thought of as a consequence of individual decision-making,[93] and individuals are expected to manage risk through their consumption and health practices.[94] Neoliberal tendencies drive contemporary public-health initiatives by touting the importance of individual risk-reducing behavior.[95] Public health today also generally emphasizes anticipating future and unintended health consequences via the "precautionary principle"[96]—the idea being that if something is *suspected* of being risky, then those risks should be avoided altogether.[97] The pre-pregnancy care model is another attempt to eradicate uncertainty in modern risk culture[98] in which individuals are preoccupied with the future and primed to take precautions to prevent or avoid risks.[99]

In medicine, too, individualized and risk-averse approaches have recently centered on advanced anticipation of risk, that is, on the practice of intervening upon potential risks that are presumed to appear in the future. For instance, scholars have focused on tendencies in contemporary medicine toward treating healthy populations as if they are primed for illness.[100] Historian Charles Rosenberg uses the examples of emergent pre-diseases, such as elevated cholesterol or pre-hypertension, to refer to "proto-disease states."[101] Pharmaceuticals target future risk as well; chemoprevention, for example, involves giving a drug (tamoxifen) to women who are deemed "high risk" for breast cancer but who are otherwise healthy and show no signs of illness.[102] Contemporary biomedical technologies serve to "control the vital processes of the body and mind," becoming "technologies of optimization,"[103] and medical jurisdiction over disease now extends to "health itself"—"it is no longer necessary to manifest symptoms to be considered ill or 'at risk.'"[104] In this way, we see an escalation of health-care interventions focusing on "pre" phases, which includes pre-pregnancy care. Indeed, the pre-pregnancy care model of risk reduction dovetails with sociological insights into how contemporary medical knowledge has diffused into lay understandings of responsibility for health more generally.

To be sure, individuals themselves are expected to optimize their health in every way possible, partially through anticipating any potential risk. This phenomenon is typified throughout the health and wellness industry; for example, employers and health insurance companies are increasingly offering financial incentives for workers to get "wellness" checks or to sign tobacco-free attestations, with the goal of assessing present and potential health risks. Current fixation with optimizing health risks is reflective of the modern biopolitical moment, one in which the "calculated management of life" works to control the behavior of both individual bodies and populations.[105] Reproductive health concerns are not atypical in this regard. Indeed, from alcohol to fish consumption, medical and public health expectations about reducing reproductive risk fill our public airwaves,[106] serving to shape and monitor behavior.

Medical sociologists have noted that this rise of "surveillance medicine," especially since the latter part of the twentieth century, has included increased medical screening and public health campaigns, conjuring the need for "anticipatory care . . . transform(ing) the future by changing the health attitudes and health behaviors of the present."[107] Anticipation is exactly what the pre-pregnancy care framework seizes upon. Reproduction and science studies scholars Vincanne Adams, Michelle Murphy, and Adele Clarke have written that "anticipation is rapidly reconfiguring technoscientific and biomedical practices as a totalizing orientation" and that "anticipation pervades the ways we think about, feel and address our contemporary problems."[108] These scholars theorize about "anticipatory regimes," in which the management of the future "requires projecting ever further back into younger years, positing the future as urgent in ever earlier moments of organismic development."[109] Additionally, exemplary sites of anticipatory regimes, according to Adams, Murphy, and Clarke, are often highly biomedical and gendered. When it comes to the next generation's health, the vector of anticipatory risk is often a woman.[110] Thus, all women of reproductive age are placed in a holding category for anticipatory care practices and interventions. In pre-pregnancy care, nonpregnant women of childbearing age are classified clinically through a framework in which the "future arrives as already formed in the present, as if the emergency has already happened."[111]

The new temporal space of pre-pregnancy risk surely is indicative of this anticipatory phenomenon in biomedicine and public health policy. Yet, pre-pregnancy risk also extends and layers previous anticipatory risk discourse in interesting and novel ways, which I elaborate upon in Chapter 3. With the zero trimester, greater levels of anticipation than have been documented exist, targeting two bodies: the potentially-pregnant woman and her future fetus. Attention and anticipation are thus partly directed toward a not-yet-conceived, non-existent being. Pre-pregnancy care can be seen as the crest of a wave of new public health and medical discourses and interventions that simultaneously focus on one present body and (at least) one future body—on the next generation through a present pre-reproductive body.

THE MATERNAL IMPERATIVE

The rise of this dual-body future emphasis is possible because of—and is characterized by—its gendered dimension. Women are typically asked to bear the burden of minimizing reproductive risk. Mothers, in particular, have long been exhorted to follow medical experts' advice about how best to raise healthy children. A hundred years ago, the medical community deployed government pamphlets and manuals to formally define proper health behavior related to pregnancy and motherhood.[112] In an example of noteworthy stasis, medical and self-care advice is still today part of the construction of contemporary "moral motherhood."[113]

The notion of the "future fetus" in the pre-pregnancy model is imaginable because of the way in which the fetus has become such a salient cultural and medical object within a surveillance society.[114] Indeed, maternal bodies get caught in a distinctive web of expert surveillance so as to optimize both fetal and infant health outcomes. Pregnant bodies today are consistently monitored to assess risks to the fetus in particular.[115] The rise of maternal-fetal medicine (MFM), fetal surgery techniques, and technoscientific practices in the second half of the twentieth century shifted obstetrical gaze toward the fetus as a separate patient, one that is distinct from the mother's body.[116] Fetal risks are often now weighed against the risks to the mother, heightening the supposed maternal-fetal conflict, in which women's interests are putatively pitted against the interests of the fetus.[117]

The rise of pre-pregnancy care thus has occurred in a climate in which maternal behavior and motherhood have higher stakes than ever before. The increased social and cultural importance placed on children[118] has much to do with this, as motherhood in general became an ever more rigorous endeavor over the course of the twentieth century. Sociologist Sharon Hays noted the rise of "intensive mothering" almost twenty years ago, referring to the idea that contemporary motherhood in the United States is labor intensive, expert driven, emotionally consuming, consumer driven, and child centered.[119] Since the time that Hays introduced her concept, mothering has intensified into what Joan B. Wolf calls "total motherhood," a concept that calls attention to the ubiquity of "risk analysis to prescriptions for good mothering in a risk culture."[120] Today, a new "momism" accentuates expectations in an increasingly idealized version of motherhood,[121] in which mothers actively engage in risk calculations on behalf of their children's health.[122]

The concepts of "intensive mothering" and "total motherhood" are helpful in gaining an understanding of contemporary messages surrounding the ever-more-diffuse health risks that are aimed at reproductively capable women. As mentioned above, in a risk culture in which individuals are expected to calculate and mitigate any potential risks,[123] and in which mothers are expected to reduce all risks to their children—especially through proper health behaviors[124]—such risk-reducing sentiments also apply to fetal health as well as to *future* fetal health. For the past several decades, "assumptions of maternal vulnerability have been reconstructed around risks to the fetus mediated through the maternal body" and even the pre-maternal body.[125] Some scholarly work has even tied the rise of the pre-pregnancy care to post-9/11 anxieties about terror, risk, and the need for increased protection of future children not yet conceived.[126]

Amplified focus on pre-pregnancy care and the rise of the zero trimester promote what I call in this book a cultural ethic of "anticipatory motherhood." Drawing on the work of Hays and Wolf, this idea positions *all* women of childbearing age as pre-pregnant and exhorts them to minimize health risks to future pregnancies, even when conception is not on the horizon. This idea is further reflective of how an American ideology of motherhood is as strong as ever, making it a persistent master status and making maternal sacrifice a master cultural frame.[127] The expectation today is that pregnancy—and thus children—can be perfected ahead of time.[128] It follows then that the rise of the pre-pregnancy care model intersects clearly with contentious reproductive politics around family planning and the changing realities of women's lives in the twenty-first century.

THE POLITICS OF MATERNAL AND
REPRODUCTIVE HEALTH

The demographics of American women's reproductive lives reveal that they are situated within the zero trimester more squarely than ever. Many women today spend years—if not decades—avoiding pregnancy.[129] Women are waiting later in life to have their first baby and are having fewer babies overall,[130] extending the so-called pre-pregnant phase to a lengthier time frame than was the case historically. Moreover, about 15% of women aged forty to forty-four report that they are childless, and this number is growing.[131] Concerns of *whether* and *when* a woman will have a baby thus potentially increase social anxiety about the expanded temporal period of women's lives when they are planning their futures. Modern views of fertility revolve around what famed demographer Ansley Coale described as a "calculus of conscious choice"[132]—that with the availability of contraception and family-planning techniques, women and couples are presumed to have the option to avoid pregnancies and to plan and space births according to their wishes. About half of the pregnancies occurring in the United States, however, still are categorized as unintended. The greater emphasis on a pre-pregnancy care framework around the turn of the twenty-first century has not been just due to prenatal care failing, as detailed already; it also is about women's increasing control over their fertility, changes in fertility patterns, and the politicized nature of reproduction and health care.

Thus, a discussion of pre-pregnancy care cannot be divorced from trends in reproductive health politics, and especially abortion politics, which grew with vehemence starting in the 1970s. As Chapter 4 elaborates, the pre-pregnancy care framework advances overlap between maternal and reproductive health—realms long considered to be separate in terms of ideology and policy—and, in so doing, strategically avoids a discussion about abortion and women's reproductive options after conception occurs. If all pregnancies are twelve-month pregnancies, then women would ostensibly have thought through their reproductive desires prior to pregnancy. The circumvention of abortion talk fits well with a broader cultural milieu that is often hostile to women's choices that do not match a maternalist or pronatalist agenda.

Studying the zero trimester by examining cultural and pregnancy risk messages that are aimed at non-pregnant women of reproductive age shows how maternal responsibility is defined for women writ large. Much reproduction scholarship looks at issues of pregnancy and fertility or focuses on women who are either already mothers or already pregnant. Social science analyses of the pre-pregnancy period mostly have concerned infertility and assisted reproductive technologies.[133] This type of analysis, however, is specifically related to women who already *desire* a baby and who are actively aspiring to conceive. This book instead analytically leverages the zero trimester—a concept that applies to all women of reproductive age, regardless of desire or capacity to get pregnant—through the lenses of reproductive risk and anticipatory motherhood. Moreover, ample human-reproduction scholarship has focused on the politics of reproduction. In this book, I more specifically deliberate the politics of reproductive risk—calling attention to the formation and deployment of discourse about the prevention of adverse reproductive outcomes.

Pregnancy and reproduction are private and individual processes, yet at the same time they also are highly visible public ones.[134] Maternal and child health outcomes proxy a nation's health and reflect on our healthcare institutions. As such, they signal some of our most pressing social issues and problems. They also reflect shifting cultural norms, such as the concerns around unintended pregnancy. Reproductive outcomes also matter intimately to individuals, especially because most women become mothers in their lifetime.[135] How women, families, physicians, and policy makers are primed to think about the risks to a healthy pregnancy is vital. One could say that, as a society, we have a generalized wish for reducing risks to pregnancy health.

The following pages document how the imperatives of prevention, concerns around the social roles of women, and the fraught politics of reproduction molded the construction of a vibrant health and policy definition of reproductive risk—one that expands medical and social control over women's bodies, from menarche to menopause, in the twenty-first century.

OVERVIEW OF THE BOOK

To understand the rise and consequences of this twenty-first century medical and social model for pregnancy health, and the zero trimester notion that accompanies it, I pursued a multisited ethnographic approach[136] and carefully examined public-health campaign documents, medical literature, policy decisions, public health reports, newsletters from maternal and child health organizations, my field notes from attendance and participation in national meetings on pre-conception health, and cultural materials such as popular advice books. For this book I also drew heavily from in-depth interviews I conducted with fifty-seven health experts who helped forge the pre-pregnancy care framework through the federal government's sponsorship. Using a "core set" method from science studies,[137] I interviewed a central group of experts—identified by the CDC as some of the top people in the field—who participated in the national meetings of the CDC's Preconception Health and Health Care Initiative in the 2000s, during which time they were charged with developing an advocacy plan for, and a definition of, pre-pregnancy care.[138] Included in these interviews were high-profile scientists, physicians, public-health experts, government health officials, and respected maternal and child health clinicians from across America.[139] Using this wide-range of sources, this book offers a nuanced story of the complex ascendance of the "zero trimester" in the United States.[140] At its heart, this book is an examination of a new way of thinking and talking about women's reproductive health—aimed at a better understanding of how current messages targeting the behaviors of reproductive-aged women came to be possible.

Focusing on the medical literature regarding pregnancy health risk from the nineteenth century to the publication of the seminal 2006 CDC *MMWR* recommendations, Chapter 2 discusses the extent to which medical thinking about the antecedents of healthy pregnancies and births has vacillated among extremes—from thinking that a woman's (or in some cases a man's) mental and physical state *during the moment of conception* is paramount, to thinking that everything a woman does *during pregnancy* matters, to thinking that everything a woman does *prior to pregnancy* is of principal importance. Pre-pregnancy risk factors were not new in the medical literature, but by the end of the twentieth century they were rearticulated by experts as a path-breaking approach to understanding reproductive risk. Hence, pre-pregnancy discourse was reframed to include myriad medical and social problems—such as pregnancy intentions—and culminated in the publication of the CDC's 2006 report.

Chapter 3 and Chapter 4 look beyond the "official" knowledge evinced in medical literature and incorporate the words and ideas of experts involved in developing and disseminating the pre-pregnancy care framework for the twenty-first century. Chapter 3 seeks to understand exactly how experts who worked with the CDC's initiative defined risks to healthy pregnancies, as well as how they thought and talked about reproductive risk and responsibility. Drawing on interviews with these experts, this chapter details how they drew on long-held notions about strong ties between women's bodies and reproductive outcomes in constructing knowledge about future risk. They also discussed the lack of robust evidence available to bolster a pre-pregnancy care model, relying instead on the facile idea that it just "makes sense" that healthier women will produce better outcomes.

Chapter 3 shows how thinking around pre-pregnancy care relied on reductionist notions of women's bodies and roles, but Chapter 4 complicates the story by showing how experts understood that framing the health of women of reproductive age in terms of pregnancy was necessarily responsive to a particular political valence. In Chapter 4, I reflect on the state of women's health care and policy that undergirds the contemporary vibrancy of the pre-pregnancy care framework. Pre-pregnancy care was in part created to advance reproductive justice by bridging the long-divided realms of maternal care and reproductive care, and in so doing avoided potential political minefields. This bridging work helped to expand women's health care during their reproductive years. The idea of couching women's health in terms of maternity status successfully followed a long tradition of maternalist policy making in America. Chapter 3 and Chapter 4 together bolster the idea that problems of knowledge are also problems of social order.[141]

Chapter 5 and Chapter 6 look at the message's roll out. Specifically, Chapter 5 details how pre-pregnancy care has been taken up clinically and culturally. In recent years, health organizations have operationalized pre-pregnancy care by using a clinical tool called the "reproductive life plan." With this questionnaire, clinicians aim to ask all women of reproductive age about their desired maternal status in the future and advise them to take precautionary action in accordance. Moreover, women's magazines and popular advice books and websites have seized on this moment.

Women and prospective parents are now inundated with information about how their reproductive years should revolve around maternity. This pre-maternal focus, I argue, betrays a neoliberal trend in which individual responsibility is paramount.

Chapter 6 analyzes how the pre-pregnancy care model has influenced public health promotion by analyzing a specific CDC campaign from 2013 called "Show Your Love." This campaign invited women of reproductive age to "show love" to their future babies, urging them to act as mothers even if they were not envisioning motherhood in their near future. In this chapter, I argue that the power of this messaging potentially changes how we think about what constitutes intensive motherhood. As is shown, this campaign—at least in its initial installment—used racialized messages that depict white women as responsible planners and women of color as "non-planners," reifying dominant tropes about the types of women who embody reproductive responsibility and thus further stratifying and racializing reproductive health.

In the concluding chapter, I reconsider the social and medical trends that have intersected with this knowledge shift in understanding pregnancy health risk. The emergence of pre-pregnancy care is about disappointment with maternal and infant health care in America, the stubbornness in thinking that links all reproductive outcomes to women's individual behaviors, and about the tendency in contemporary medicine and public health toward the anticipation of risk. But it is also about our inability in the United States to consider abortion within a comprehensive and responsible discussion about reproductive health; it is about the rising medical and political visibility of the fetus, our growing desire to perfect pregnancies, the rise of anticipatory motherhood, and social and medical concerns about women's changing life-course patterns.

The public-health messages highlighted at the beginning of this chapter are different from a decades-long medical and public health focus on the nine months of pregnancy. The focus is today, rather and decidedly, on the zero trimester—on the non-pregnant woman's body and future motherhood status. The growing sentiment that women should improve their pre-pregnancy health to reduce reproductive risk is part of broader medical and cultural tendencies toward focusing on the pre-pregnancy health of women. The rise of the "zero trimester" is not simply about medical and health concerns; it is more broadly about struggles and entanglements over the cultural power and social ideologies that shape women's bodily experiences and population-health imperatives.

On a final introductory note, it is perhaps necessary to emphasize that, over the course of this research, I have struggled with respect to whether I regard the pre-pregnancy care model as "good" or "bad" for women. I am sympathetic with critiques that claim the model is "dangerous for women," and I highlight many instances in this book where I believe this to be so. And yet, through speaking with many experts and following this topic over time, I understand that the pre-pregnancy care model is one that hinges on reproductive-justice notions of expanded health services for all women, regardless of whether they eventually become mothers. This book does not provide a conclusive answer as to whether the model is backward and reductionist or progressive and liberating. It is complicated, and it is probably both.

This book rather aims to highlight the historical, cultural, and political underpinnings of pre-pregnancy care, embracing instead of eschewing all the nuances that come with such an analysis. The concluding chapter returns to questions of how, going forward, we might think with, around, and beyond this model in reproductive health. The intervening chapters offer empirical findings that upend conventional wisdom on both sides of the debate while offering an argument that pre-pregnancy care is neither wholly hostile to feminist progress nor the saving grace for women and babies in America. At the very least, the rise of the "zero trimester" does mean that notions of womanhood and motherhood are intertwined as much as ever before, if not more so.

2 From the Womb to the Woman

THE SHIFTING LOCUS OF REPRODUCTIVE RISK

Much twenty-first-century literature covering the pre-pregnancy care model dates its emergence to a 1980 publication in the *British Medical Journal*. In the article, physician Geoffrey Chamberlain called for a "pre-pregnancy clinic" to give women "authoritative advice" concerning future pregnancies.[1] Although publication of this article proved to be a critical event in the medical establishment's recognition of pre-pregnancy care, it was not nearly the beginning of its history.

Identifying the factors that pose risks to a healthy pregnancy is a timeless concern, one that has long consumed social thought and that has long vexed the medical community. Ideas about how women's or men's characteristics or behaviors might impact reproductive outcomes have existed since at least classical antiquity,[2] and it is clear even in classical texts that the importance of general reproductive health to the health of future generations was of paramount import. More than 2,500 years ago, for example, Plutarch was concerned with the health of young Spartan women and girls. For fear that they might otherwise endanger the quality of future reproduction, he wrote that "maidens" should make sure to exercise "to the end that the fruit they conceived might, in strong and healthy bodies, take firmer root and find better growth."[3]

In the twentieth century, the reproductive factors that dominated medical and policy focus on birth outcomes were clustered *during the period of pregnancy*—and prenatal care was the medical intervention of choice for ensuring healthy pregnancy outcomes. Despite the overwhelming focus on the prenatal period in recent history, the reproductive phase on which medical investigation centers actually has been quite variable over time. Periodically, concerns about reducing risks to healthy pregnancies have focused intently on factors in the pre-pregnancy period. This chapter traces the evolution of health professionals' thinking about how medicine and public health should intervene to ensure healthy pregnancies, focusing specifically on the extent to which medical thought has implicated pre-pregnancy health and health care as influencing reproductive outcomes. Reflecting on medical literature from the nineteenth century through the end of the twentieth century, this chapter reveals how physicians have highlighted the pre-pregnancy period with varying intensity and degree over time.[4]

The idea of "pre-pregnancy care" did not begin in 1980, and such contemporary proclamations that claim otherwise miss an unsavory history. Assertions about pre-pregnancy health have existed for millennia, but pre-pregnancy *care* emerged in the medical literature in the early twentieth century as a concerted strategy to facilitate eugenics-minded medicine as well as to battle syphilis. These two historical moments are highlighted in this chapter as instances when the pre-pregnancy care of women—and often men—was organized. Any other focus on pre-pregnancy health and health care largely was overshadowed in the twentieth century by the rising focus on factors in the womb and on prenatal care. As sociologist Elizabeth M. Armstrong has written, the locus of reproductive risk in the twentieth century was indeed the womb; *in utero* became the frame of choice in medical and scientific investigations into the causes of reproductive outcomes.[5] The demise of prenatal care as a truly preventive tool in the eyes of health professionals by the late twentieth century, along with demographic and political shifts related to childbearing and women's reproductive lives, caused pre-pregnancy discourse to resurge in the medical literature—in many ways shifting the locus of risk for a healthy pregnancy from the womb to the woman.

HEALTHY PREGNANCY IN THE
NINETEENTH CENTURY

Fetal development was not well understood in the nineteenth century, yet there were widely held beliefs about certain factors that might put a pregnancy in peril. One dominant trope during this time was the doctrine of maternal impressions—a theory that specifically situated the cause of congenital malformations in the mental and emotional experiences of the mother while she was pregnant. In the *New England Journal of Medicine and Surgery* in 1824, for example, one doctor retold a story of a woman being frightened during pregnancy by a large tortoise near her house; she subsequently gave birth to a "misshapen mass."[6] Accounts such as this one often referred to the fetus as a grotesque creature, as in 1829 when an Ohio physician wrote to the *Boston Medical and Surgical Journal* to report that he delivered a premature "monster"—one that resembled a puppy—from a woman who was frightened early in her pregnancy by two fighting dogs.[7] No medical care could ensure that a pregnant woman did not experience a social situation that might "mark" her child; rather, these kinds of stories in the professional literature served as a form of speculation about the root cause of birth defects. Pregnant women were simply told to avoid risks to their emotional state as much as possible. Maternal impressions thus constituted a theory that resonated with ideas at the time that attributed successful pregnancies to a balanced lifestyle,[8] tying together the vicissitudes of daily social life with medical outcomes.

In the early part of the nineteenth century, the fetus and eventual infant were considered "malleable" until the child was weaned. Yet medical assumptions about the transmission of traits often led both popular and scientific thought to focus on the quality of the moment of conception[9]—an emphasis neither on pre-pregnancy nor on pregnancy but rather on the health status of both parents while conceiving. Couples were urged to be of good nature during intercourse, or else the subsequent offspring might be harmed. The pregnant woman was told then to exhibit loving and gracious qualities so as to ensure the health and the morality of the fetus.[10] It was not until the middle of the nineteenth century that "heredity" as a formal concept emerged as a prominent piece of both medical explanation and social thought.[11] Birth defects and birth outcomes were rather mostly understood during this time as results of the state of emotions either in the pregnant woman, in the case of maternal impressions, or in both parents, as in the focus on the health of the conception.

Still, there was plenty of medical and social thought that centered on factors visible well *before* conception ever took place. In fact, although much prevailing medical thinking about heredity in the nineteenth century assumed that it was the exact moment of conception that conferred the "biological identities of both parents," those identities were defined as "resultants of the cumulative interaction of all those habits, accidents, illnesses—and original constitutional endowments—which had *intersected since their own conception.*"[12] Twenty-first century epigenetics explanations of birth and life outcomes do not sound all that dissimilar from this sentiment. The nineteenth-century theory of diathesis focused on individual predispositions to disease as part of one's constitutional makeup over a lifetime. For example, the offspring of someone who consumes alcohol was assumed to inherit not only the propensity to drink but also a certain "package of constitutional weaknesses."[13] That is, individuals' life histories and general temperaments—those of both women and men—were highlighted as mattering for the health of future offspring. These theories and discussions largely did not implicate the need for medical care; rather, women and men were simply urged to lead proper and moral lifestyles to ensure the health of their reproductive futures.

Nevertheless, much medical emphasis specifically was placed on women and on the surveillance of women's social behaviors. In one of the first American textbooks on pediatrics, William Potts Dewees in 1825 wrote that "the physical treatment of children should begin as far as may be practicable, with the earliest formation of the embryo; it will, therefore, necessarily involve the conduct of the mother, *even before her marriage*, as well as during her pregnancy."[14] This quote includes not only concern about ensuring the health of future children but also about the mother's moral conduct. Indeed, throughout the nineteenth century, claims were made about limiting women's social engagement for the very purpose of "protecting" their future reproductive bodies. Dr. Edward Hammond Clarke's 1873 treatise, *Sex in Education*,[15] set off a political firestorm as he claimed that women who pursued higher education would suffer reproductive debilities.[16] Experts thus argued that women's future pregnancies would be endangered lest they abide social conventions of the time. These messages, of course, were mostly directed at white women in America, as black women had long been regarded as important reproducers but in a very different way in terms of the future of the nation. Although children born of slaves were deemed necessary for the depraved fabric of the antebellum economy, slave women were not treated in a way that "protected their future" in any manner of the phrase.[17]

In the nineteenth century, physicians generally saw (white) women as "the product and prisoner of her reproductive system."[18] As such, women increasingly sought to limit their fertility through a variety of means; "potential mothers" also were castigated for their role in "race suicide."[19] To ensure the vitality of future reproductive endeavors, women were asked to do everything from exercising routinely to dressing appropriately. In a medical journal article on breastfeeding, for example, one physician wrote that "before pregnancy and even before marriage women ought to be taught to admire this really most beautiful function of woman-hood. Girls should be taught to guard their breasts and nipples from the injury false fashions of dress impose."[20] All of women's reproductive functions and body parts were under surveillance in the pre-pregnancy period—or, to use the euphemism of the time, in the "pre-marriage period"—in the service of the health and purported decency of future generations.

If a woman experienced poor reproductive outcomes, then it was assumed that she had lived a pre-pregnant lifestyle not conducive with healthful reproduction. In another 1824 article in the *New England Journal of Medicine and Surgery*, a physician recounted an experience with a woman who had an early spontaneous abortion. Reporting that "her health was not very good at any time, and had not improved during her pregnancy,"[21] the physician explained that to treat a spontaneous abortion is also to treat "the patient before a second conception"—that is, in this physician's view, the times between reproductive events blended together and should be seen as preventive care in preparation for the next (healthier) time.[22] The nineteenth-century medical literature was peppered with these types of assessments of general pre-pregnancy health and ideas about how to intervene medically. Physicians were puzzled when healthy women experienced poor reproductive outcomes, tying such events to lifestyle and moral behavior.

In another medical article on spontaneous abortion, for example, a physician tried to explain how such an event could happen in women who seem otherwise very healthy. The physician attributed spontaneous abortion to life choices that were made in the pre-pregnancy phase, arguing that sometimes these women "are married late in life; have been luxurious livers . . . [and] have good health."[23] The physician conjectured that this variety of abortion belongs to a type in which "the general health is too good for healthy pregnancy."[24] In this appraisal, top-notch pre-pregnancy health actually could be detrimental—some white women's life of luxury had not situated them well for motherhood, but it was all in the service of expositing what was deemed "proper" pre-pregnancy lifestyles. Physicians thus were clearly enamored with women's lifestyle choices such as age at marriage and first pregnancy—likening any desires that deviated from early marriage and motherhood as potentially damaging to their future reproductive outcomes.

Physicians also were interested in whether certain physiological reproductive risks were present during the pre-pregnancy period. In 1887, writing about a rare case of a pregnancy taking place within a uterus that had structural abnormalities, a physician discussed the patient's reproductive history prior to her pregnancy and emphasized the idea that the uterine position was likely laterally flexed *prior to pregnancy*, which of course was not diagnosed prior to the pregnancy.[25] In accounts of Bright's disease from the same time, physicians accentuated that having the condition prior to pregnancy exacerbated the seriousness of disease during pregnancy.[26] Similarly, the cause of a case of puerperal eclampsia was "probably from an endometriosis existing prior to conception."[27] In 1895, in a piece on metritis (inflammation of uterine wall) as a cause of miscarriage, a physician highlighted that treatments might be best before pregnancy, writing, "As to the treatment, I may say at once that it is very difficult to treat an endometritis as long as pregnancy is going on. The only good practice is the preventive treatment which is undertaken when the uterine cavity is empty in cases in which an inflammation of the uterine mucosa has occurred *before the pregnancy* or when it has already produced miscarriages."[28] In many of these instances, physicians mentioned how pre-pregnancy care might have helped the woman's circumstances, but there was no organized idea about proper medical care prior to conception.

Pre-pregnancy health discussions were rather mostly reflective of general concerns over women's social behaviors leading up to marriage and motherhood as well as speculations about physiological abnormalities prior to pregnancy that might pose medical risks to a woman's reproductive capacity and future reproductive outcomes. Discussions over venereal diseases serve as good examples of just how intermingled were the worlds of social concern and medical concern, of social policy and ideas about reproductive health care interventions. The following section briefly considers the prolific medical literature on syphilis as illustrative.

VENEREAL DISEASE AS AN EARLY HUB OF PRE-PREGNANCY DISCOURSE

Syphilis was a public-health menace around the turn of the twentieth century. A common topic in the medical literature regarding the potential health of future offspring, syphilis was usually discussed vis-à-vis social and moral interventions as well as medical interventions. One article by Abner Post in an 1889 issue of the *Boston Medical and Surgical Journal* was titled "Some Considerations Concerning Syphilis and Marriage" and asked the question of whether two syphilitics should marry and, by extension, reproduce. For the man in question, Post's answer was that nothing would be worsened because he was already syphilitic, but for the woman the concern was about future pregnancies. Post's answer to syphilitic couples wanting to conceive was to wait until they experience two full years of symptom-free living, at which point he also prescribed a course of mercury treatment before conception.[29] Dr. Post's recommendation served as an early example of a precise pre-pregnancy medical intervention.

In 1912, the article "Epitome of Current Medical Literature" in the *British Medical Journal* discussed a case of syphilis in terms of its "conceptional" basis, highlighting the prophylactic promise of "preconceptional treatment" with regard to syphilis to produce "healthy children and to avoid conceptional infection of the wife."[30] In one of the first medical mentions of a pre-pregnancy "treatment regime," the focus remained on *both* the maternal and paternal influences on the quality of the conceptus. In fact, much of the literature on syphilis focused on men and their responsibilities. Many physicians in the nineteenth century accepted Colles's Law, which posited that syphilis was passed from sperm to fetus, completely bypassing the mother.[31]

The pre-pregnancy discussions around syphilis and other "conditions" were concerned mostly with leading a "proper lifestyle" and with social concerns endemic to the pre-pregnancy period, such as marital fidelity or the spread of sexually transmitted disease. In his history of venereal disease, historian Allan Brandt notes that "these themes had particular resonance for American physicians, who were already concerned about the future of the family."[32] Many physicians during this time who were concerned about how venereal diseases were impacting the family allied with the eugenics movement, seeing venereal diseases as impacting the future of "the race."[33] Indeed, declining birth rates of whites were seen as a sign of the demise of American values, and reproductive matters were front and center not only for public health purposes but also for population concerns. Many states passed "eugenic marriage laws" whereby only the prospective husband had to undergo a physician assessment and "receive a certification of health"[34] before getting married and thus, presumably, before procreating. Near the turn of the twentieth century, physicians thus believed it was in their province—as both medical and moral leaders—to advise patients against entering into "hasty marriages."[35]

Thomas Parran, surgeon general under Franklin Delano Roosevelt, further sought to make venereal disease a national concern, and pre-pregnancy interventions were at the forefront of his agenda. One of Parran's suggestions included mandatory blood tests prior to marriage as well as in early pregnancy.[36] Beginning with Connecticut in 1935, as Brandt recounts, in many states a premarital blood test became a standard requirement for a couple prior to obtaining a marriage license.[37] In Connecticut in particular, if either the bride or groom was found to be infected, the couple had to wait—sometime years—before procuring a marriage license, until the said individual was found to be infection free,[38] a process that certainly reflected government surveillance of the pre-pregnancy period. By 1938, twenty-six states had provisions on the books prohibiting the marriage of infected individuals.[39] Marriage, of course, was the assumed precursor to reproduction during this time. To regulate women's and men's bodies in the pre-pregnancy phase was to regulate marriage.

Not all the attention in syphilis campaigns was focused on the pre-pregnancy period or on unmarried men and women. Pregnant women also came under surveillance. In 1938, New York and Rhode Island enacted laws requiring prenatal blood tests to check for syphilis, and these laws spread across the United States.[40] As Brandt documents, early and continuous treatment of syphilis in pregnancy worked, and these laws had a significant public-health impact: infant mortality rates from syphilis dropped precipitously.[41] Although public-health messages regarding syphilis targeted the pre-pregnancy period and social activities such as marriage, it was actually treatment during pregnancy that turned out to be most successful. The syphilis example shows that while pre-pregnancy messages functioned as a social policy tool, medical treatment during pregnancy had the most demonstrable effect for such a specific problem as syphilis. This outcome helped propel prenatal care as the gold-standard for pregnancy health care during the twentieth century. Telling citizens what to do during the pre-pregnancy period was not found to be helpful for the most part. That is, attempting primary prevention did not work in this instance. Treatment with pregnancy care—rather than prevention, with pre-pregnancy care—emerged as the typical way to think about disease and reproductive outcomes. Pre-pregnancy care was shifted further to the margins of medical discussions about reproductive risk.

Indeed, treatment for syphilis and preeclampsia surfaced in the medical literature in the early twentieth century as model cases for the need for *prenatal* interventions in high-risk pregnancies. As such, focus trended away from pre-pregnancy and lifestyle factors as prenatal care gained prominence, along with the attendant assumption that medical care would fix pregnancy problems. Pre-pregnancy care messages began to be eclipsed by prenatal care discussions. Up until the rise of prenatal care, pre-pregnancy health often was discussed as either something women should maintain (through proper dress and education) or something that was out of women's control (their pre-pregnancy reproductive tract problems) or simply as a man's fault (with syphilis). Yet, over time, pre-pregnancy health increasingly became something of a woman's domain, something that was highlighted as within her purview to control and preserve. Medical care increasingly became less about high-risk pregnancies (say, a syphilitic pregnant woman) and more about optimizing every single pregnancy, no matter its risk status. This shift toward greater maternal responsibility along with expanded prenatal care to populations not necessary "at risk" largely was an outgrowth of the shift in focus toward pregnancy behaviors—on prenatal care and on the womb—that dominated medical literature of the twentieth century.

THE ADVENT OF PRENATAL CARE

No formal care mechanism was in place for pregnant women in the nineteenth century. For the most part, women did not seek medical care during their pregnancies; there were few hospitals or offices where pregnancy care took place; the concept of "prenatal care" did not even exist.[42] To achieve a successful pregnancy or birth outcome did not involve seeking medical attention throughout one's pregnancy. There were some prenatal therapies available (such as bloodletting or abdominal palpation), should a woman present to a physician during pregnancy with a risky situation, but most clinical intervention for pregnant women in the nineteenth century was focused on lifestyle advice,[43] just as it was for pre-pregnant women.

At the turn of the twentieth century, doctors began more seriously to identify factors that could harm a fetus *in utero* rather than contemplating effects prior to pregnancy. A good example of this is found in a 1907 *British Medical Journal* article on the "Unborn Child," in which a gynecologist wrote that, "Although, as a matter of fact, *the deepest foundations are laid long before conception*, the future health and constitution of the child are intimately bound up with the processes which go on *during its intrauterine existence*."[44] In this article, the "rights" of the unborn are enumerated, which include the recognition that parents should provide "a clean and normal life before and after conception,"[45] but the growing emphasis in medicine was on the womb during pregnancy.

The organized clinical monitoring and treatment of pregnant women as we know prenatal care to be today usually is traced to an article published in the *British Medical Journal* in 1901. In his "Plea for a Pro-Maternity Hospital," physician J. W. Ballantyne wrote about the need for a distinct area in the Maternity Hospital that would "be for the reception of women who are pregnant but who are not yet in labour."[46] He was focused on preventing "morbid pregnancy," and wrote about the importance of prenatal care for advancing preventive medicine more broadly.[47]

It remained curious to medical professionals at the time why otherwise healthy women would give birth to a baby with abnormalities or why she or the infant might die in childbirth. Although there were no conclusive data that expanding prenatal care would work to offset these risks—in fact, prenatal care services were usually included as part of lists of suspected *causes* of maternal or infant mortality[48]—prenatal care was constructed as the primary *solution* to infant mortality and morbidity.[49] When prenatal care was first practiced in England in the early twentieth century, protocols did not refer to the early pregnancy period but rather began instruction around the fourth or fifth month and consisted mainly of urine analysis and general advice.[50] In England, by the 1920s, prenatal care was considered the cure for all reproductive ailments.[51] Prenatal care had begun its ascent as the presumed magic bullet for reducing reproductive risk in the twentieth century.

This belief in the promise of prenatal care was also emergent in the United States. During the first two decades of the twentieth century in the United States, numerous labor protections and social regulations were legislated by states and by Congress to "help adult American women as mothers or *as potential mothers*."[52] The Children's Bureau, started in 1912, began promoting prenatal care in 1913.[53] In 1921, the Sheppard-Towner Maternity and Infancy Protection Act passed as the first major welfare program in the United States and was partly concerned with providing prenatal care to pregnant women. Prenatal care thus constituted part of a major policy and medical thrust in the early twentieth century. As a result, the overwhelming focus of discussions about pregnancy health risk in the early to middle part of the twentieth century was on prenatal factors.[54]

Soon, however, individuals began questioning what exactly prenatal care was achieving. As Ann Oakley documents in England, the chief goal of prenatal care was to reduce risks of pregnancy and childbearing for the mother, but results on this front were not moving forward and were characterized as "obscure and perplexing."[55] By the 1930s, physicians began looking for reasons for the "failure" of prenatal care[56]: "Supervision at an antenatal clinic will not by itself save life."[57] Years earlier, Ballantyne himself had gestured to the necessity of pre-pregnancy services in addition to the prenatal ones. In a review of his influential work *Manual of Antenatal Pathology and Hygiene: The Embryo,*[58] the *British Medical Journal* noted that Ballantyne's concluding chapter covers how "the *preconceptional* period of germinal life is identical with morbid heredity."[59]

In a similar vein, a popular nursing text stated, in 1929, that prenatal care should begin "perhaps even earlier" than when a patient conceives.[60] In a 1934 combined meeting between obstetrics/gynecology and public health, experts reviewed the state of prenatal care. One of the doctors was quoted as claiming that *preconception* care "was almost more important than ante-natal care," as the "best hope of progress lay in those agencies which were dealing with the health of growing girls."[61]

Indeed, while prenatal care was on the rise and gaining policy traction—as it would continue to do throughout the twentieth century—the medical literature did not ignore pre-pregnancy factors completely, especially in high-risk cases or in cases shrouded in uncertainty. As one physician contemplated the effects of uterine fibroids, "In general, if a fibroid is to be regarded as a menace to life before pregnancy, the condition must be still more grave after conception occurs. Is it not the duty of the gynecologist to ward off this danger?"[62] In the *New England Journal of Medicine,* speculation about spontaneous abortion continued to call attention to the pre-pregnancy period: "Preconceptional treatment may be directed toward correcting defects in the germ cells (sperm or ovum), toward the elimination of certain pelvic abnormalities and toward the treatment of systemic factors that tend to abortion."[63]

Physicians kept highlighting the pre-pregnancy period, but because treatment during pregnancy was increasingly considered the crucial medical tool for reducing reproductive risk—despite rumblings that it was doing nothing of the sort—discussions about pre-pregnancy health were often aimed at lamenting women's lifestyle choices or general health status. That is, without medical or policy backing, physicians simply took to conjecturing about women's health status before pregnancy. For example, with regard to preeclampsia, the following appeared in the *New England Journal of Medicine*: "It would, of course, be better to have the patient in the best physical condition *before pregnancy occurred.*"[64] Hypertension, in another instance, was thought to be better controlled with attention prior to pregnancy, "by the combined and co-ordinated efforts of the internist and the

obstetrician and of medical and maternity clinics, or by the constant observation and study of obstetric patients *before, during and for years after their
childbearing careers* by the physicians who attend them. . . ."[65]

Pre-pregnancy health and health-care discussions continued in the
medical literature, although they came to be somewhat marginal as compared to the prominent literature on prenatal care. Yet, the discussions
were couched in the language of social concerns and, as such, much of the
pre-pregnancy medical literature was not concerned with reducing reproductive risk per se but rather with preventing certain pregnancies in the
first place. That is to say that, in the early twentieth century, pre-pregnancy health and health care discussions became mired in population
health goals of the day, namely eugenics.

PRE-PREGNANCY HEALTH DISCOURSE AND
POPULATION CONTROL

In 1936, obstetrician Fred Adair wrote in the *Journal of the American
Medical Association* that obstetrics education should include pre-pregnancy
care knowledge.[66] In 1940, Adair, a professor of obstetrics and gynecology
at the University of Chicago, wrote one of the earliest articles to be titled
"preconceptional care."[67] He started off the article defining "preconceptional care" as, "designed to assist in securing perfect reproduction. It rests
upon fundamental eugenic and euthenic principles. It is that care and
attention which is given prior to conception and involves the elimination of
those individuals who are not suitable for wholesome reproduction and the
seduction of those who are capable of normal reproduction."[68]

Adair's statement here was in vogue with the medical literature on
eugenics. He went on to discuss the necessity of codifying a "preconceptional viewpoint" via state control of reproduction, as his state of Illinois
did in 1937 when it required potential marriage partners to be tested for
venereal disease. Indeed, although the eugenics movement was beginning
to wane in the United States in the 1930s, many U.S. states passed sterili-
zation laws clearly targeting individuals for eugenic purposes.[69] Racial
hygiene logic was part of a broad push in the United States for "better
breeding," which did not end when Nazism fell.[70]

One of the earliest mentions of the term "preconception care" came in the meeting minutes of the 1932 Annual Sessions of the American Medical Association.[71] The section on obstetrics, gynecology, and abdominal surgery was called to order by its chairman, Fred Adair, and the first paper read was on "preconceptional and prenatal care," by Percy W. Toombs of Tennessee.[72] In 1923, the *Journal of Heredity* had published a lecture by Toombs on "parenthood and race culture."[73] In this talk, Toombs outlined the aims of eugenics. His language is unsettling as a precursor to a "pre-pregnancy care framework" in the United States. He wrote, for example, that "there is a constant tendency toward relative and absolute sterility among that class of society which is best fitted to produce the next generation, and the most prolific are the less fit to carry on the torch of civilization."[74] Pre-pregnancy care discussions in the medical literature in the early twentieth century were riddled with discussions expressive of eugenic ideologies.

Remnants of pre-pregnancy care's relationship with eugenics were still found in the 1960s,[75] but this early history is erased in contemporary pre-pregnancy health and health care literature. For example, by positioning the pre-pregnancy care model as beginning with Chamberlain's U.K. clinics in 1980, as many present-day publications do, articles avoid the ways in which pre-pregnancy care was tied up with unsavory medical ideas in the earlier part of the century. Even when contemporary publications go back further than Chamberlain's article—for example, a March of Dimes publication in 2002 stated that pre-pregnancy care dates to the 1960s—they don't go back far enough.[76] Some articles cite the Dewees pediatrics textbook from the nineteenth century or even Plutarch when they mention medical concerns about pre-pregnancy *health*, but then gloss ahead to the 1980s when highlighting the beginning of pre-pregnancy *care*,[77] eliding pre-pregnancy care advocates' earlier connection with eugenics. Pre-pregnancy health and health care ideas in the first half of the twentieth century often intersected with strategies of population control, strongly linked to eugenics.

A related strain of early pre-pregnancy care literature, also stemming from obstetrics, was used to talk about family planning more broadly. At a meeting of the Southern Medical Association's section on obstetrics in 1939, one doctor argued that "preconceptional care" should be the preferred term over "birth control" because physicians are not trying to control births, but rather conception.[78] Speakers at the Southern Conference on Tomorrow's Children in 1939, which included remarks from Margaret Sanger, preferred the term "preconceptional care" to "birth control" when discussing contraceptive practices.[79]

Often, in this realm, pre-pregnancy health discussions had little to do with medical concerns directly and more to do with social concerns regarding pregnancy intentions and preventing unwanted pregnancies. This focus was strengthened by one of the most important advances in women's health care in the twentieth century: the FDA approval of the birth control pill in 1960. The notion of "family planning" also was gaining prominence. As part of President Johnson's War on Poverty, the federal government issued its first grants in support of family planning practices in 1965. In 1970, Congress enacted Title X of the Public Health Service Act to ensure family planning access for low-income women.[80] Abortion was legalized at the federal level in 1973. This policy history emerged largely separate from that of pregnancy and prenatal services mentioned above, cutting a political hole in women's health care in the United States between services for preventing pregnancies and services for safeguarding pregnancies, a point which is revisited in greater detail in Chapter 4.

Along with the growing popularity of family planning, further advances in infertility treatments and genetic screening initiated an unprecedented ability to control conception (and birth), and the idea of "planning" could thus be systematized in the latter half of the twentieth century. As demographers theorized, reproduction came to be seen during this time as increasingly under individuals' control.[81] Physicians wanted part of this control. Thus, the medical literature subsequently began to pay concerted attention to planning pregnancies with the availability of effective contraceptive technologies. Pre-pregnancy health discourse at this historical juncture in many ways became predicated on the notion of "intendedness," as physicians argued that they could more easily monitor patients and pregnancies if those pregnancies were planned—and, by extension, solve the problems of adverse birth outcomes. One obstetrician wrote that "prenatal care can be simply a system of observations, and the observation of a patient . . . prevents nothing."[82] Another physician wrote, "Since the advent of reliable methods of contraception . . . women not only expect to plan, but even to time, their pregnancies. Under these circumstances, it becomes quite feasible to advise patients to see their doctor before they expect to start a pregnancy" to "influence the events in the periconceptional period."[83]

As eugenics discourse became an abomination and the pill became popular, pre-pregnancy care discussions within the medical literature were no longer couched in the language of "better breeding" but rather of reproductive control and advising women that they should consult a doctor before getting pregnant. Crucially, this was also a time of upheaval for the profession of obstetrics.[84] Because doctors were beginning to grasp the inadequacies of prenatal care as early as the 1960s,[85] the intersection of family planning and new moments of surveillance—namely of the pre-pregnancy period—became a site for new claims of professional jurisdiction.

THE FIRST PRE-PREGNANCY CLINICS

Prior to the mid-twentieth century, mentions of care prior to conception in the medical literature focused on discussions of heredity, eugenics, and treatment of physiological and social problems that might pose risk to a healthy pregnancy. By and large, the literature was not focused on extending a formal medical model such as prenatal care to the pre-pregnancy period. In the 1950s, however, medical articles emerged that indicated some obstetricians—especially in the United States—were trying to address adverse birth outcomes through preventive pre-pregnancy care. For example, medical articles detailed a select few "fetal salvage" initiatives that were operated through "preconceptional" treatment clinics.[86] These early clinics actually focused on *inter-pregnancy* care; that is, they admitted parents who had experienced a previous adverse birth or pregnancy outcome to learn more about conception, implantation, and fetal growth prior to another pregnancy. A physician in a New York clinic explained—without offering any evidence or data—that therapies were not effective once pregnancy had begun.[87] Indeed, in this early literature, "evidence" was not used in making claims for pre-pregnancy clinics. The arguments revolved around increased management of the woman, to help the obstetrician figure out what was going wrong. One obstetrician wrote of a "preconception" clinic: "In preconceptional care the effort should be to investigate families with a history of pregnancy wastage in the interval between pregnancy, to delve deeper into the realms of environmental pathology, and to increase research in the role that endometrial insufficiency and uterine anomalies play in pregnancy wastage."[88]

In 1961, a "preconceptional regimen" was discussed to address abnormalities in fetuses.[89] In 1962, in the Chairman's Address to the section on obstetrics and gynecology at the Annual Meeting of the American Medical Association (AMA) in Chicago, the profession was called upon to care for women throughout their life—"from preconception therapy in infertility to geriatric gynecology"—or, "from the womb to the tomb."[90]

References to pre-pregnancy care were being used in myriad ways during this time. Pre-pregnancy care served as a justification when obstetrics started making a case for expanded jurisdiction into more preventive services.[91] The profession always saw prenatal care as a preventive service, but some in the field wanted to do more. The chairman of the obstetrics section of AMA argued, "This, then, such as it is, is the chairman's address—a plea for the development within ourselves of the 'Compleat Obstetrician,' no longer a mere midwife glorified as a specialist, but rather a fully rounded figure of stature in the mural that is medicine."[92] This claim was meant to argue for enhanced medical status for obstetrician-gynecologists. A similar discussion around prevention would emerge in years to come as it became clear to many obstetricians that prenatal care did not constitute active prevention but rather simply was surveillance.

A principal article in which the claims for pre-pregnancy care presaged the kinds of claims we hear today was published in 1966.[93] In the "Medical News" section of *JAMA*, "pre-pregnancy plans" were deemed the "key" to reducing infant mortality. Several obstetricians are quoted in this article as explaining that prenatal care "is not enough." The *JAMA* piece made the first elaborate claims of expanding obstetrical practice: "Programs which depend upon identification of the high risk patient early in pregnancy, combined with intensive prenatal care, are not likely to materially reduce the U.S. infant mortality rate. By the time a woman is pregnant, the risk has already been compounded."[94] The article cited a "trend" toward preconceptional and inter-conceptional care within obstetrics.

In 1970, a Canadian obstetrician-gynecologist made an argument for the logical extension of obstetrical practice into pre-pregnancy care.[95] In this article, Dr. Rhinehart Friesen called "pre-pregnancy care" a "logical extension of prenatal care" and revealed developments in embryology showing that "it is becoming increasingly apparent" that by four to six weeks post-fertilization, and before a woman usually presents at the physician's office, critical fetal development has occurred:

> by this time (four to six weeks after fertilization) the fetus has already passed the most critical period in its development. Furthermore, the effects of various noxious influences on the germ cells before fertilization cannot be nullified by earlier prenatal care. Obviously, exhortations for earlier and earlier prenatal care are not the answer to the problems presented by the dangers of the last few weeks before conception and the first all-important weeks after this event. If anything is to be done to influence the events in the periconceptional period, *probably the most dangerous time in any individual's lifetime*, it must be done before, rather than after, the woman thinks she is pregnant.[96]

The obstetrical project in the twentieth century worked to pathologize pregnancy and birth. As Arney writes in his analysis of the obstetrical profession, "obstetricians had to develop ways to 'foresee' pathology and act prophylactically because they could not always depend on pathology being obviously present."[97] Friesen's "logical" argument, as he posited it, was important because it positioned the need for obstetrical focus to cover the period around conception, thus presumably preempting any potential pathology—that is, to intervene upon, as he described the period around conception, "the most dangerous time in any individual's lifetime." Friesen argued for a pre-pregnancy visit to occur three months before discontinuing a contraceptive,[98] which lent early credence to the "twelve-month pregnancy" idea that would be promulgated by the March of Dimes and others at the end of the twentieth century.

From the 1950s to the 1970s, the pre-pregnancy medical discussions about expanding care and clinics largely were enamored with intensifying the obstetrical management of high-risk pregnancies, which were usually defined during this time as the experience of a previous adverse birth outcome. This clinical discussion, for the most part, thus was about "high-risk women" and inter-pregnancy care—a method that targets a specific group of women who have experienced a prior negative outcome (e.g., spontaneous abortion, birth defect), not every woman of reproductive age. This would soon all start to change through a U.K. pediatrician's research on folic acid and birth defects.

THE CRUCIAL ROLE OF FOLIC ACID

The folic acid studies of the 1970s and 1980s marked a critical juncture in the historical trajectory of pre-pregnancy care discussions in the medical literature.[99] In 1976, a study led by the pediatrician Richard Smithells in the United Kingdom proposed a relationship between vitamin deficiencies, particularly folate, and NTDs (neural tube defects).[100] Historian Salim Al-Gailani notes that with the launch of a clinical trial in 1977, Smithells started to transform folic acid from a routine prenatal supplement for reducing the risk of anemia into an experimental drug to reduce neural-tube birth defects in so-called "high-risk" mothers.[101] Smithells' first clinical trials were for "high-risk" women during their inter-pregnancy period—that is, the trials targeted women who had had previous adverse birth outcomes, not all women of reproductive age. The findings were published in 1980 in the *Lancet* and suggested that folic acid taken around the time of conception could reduce the risk of recurrent NTDs by half.[102] Smithells argued that this intervention was exemplary of primary prevention, better than the secondary prevention achieved through prenatal care and screening.[103] Yet, as folic acid was gaining popularity as a routine prenatal supplement, clinicians pushed back on prescribing folic acid to all pregnant women as a "blanket policy," arguing that it masked attention to the real social problems of nutrition deficiencies.[104]

Amid contested findings and ongoing discussions about widespread folic acid supplementation throughout the 1980s,[105] another randomized clinical trial, known as the U.K. Medical Research Council (MRC) study, was published in 1991 in the *Lancet*. The MRC study revealed that when women took folic acid supplementation before pregnancy, the risk of NTDs could be reduced.[106] This finding led the CDC in the United States to issue a broad recommendation for women to supplement their diet with folic acid *prior to pregnancy* for the purpose of reducing NTDs.[107] Also within months of the 1991 publication, food manufacturers initiated plans to fortify breakfast cereals; the Kellogg Company introduced a strategy to market products to "women of childbearing age" so that "babies benefit from a healthy breakfast even before they're conceived."[108] Folic acid, once intended for only high-risk individuals, became a population health strategy for all women of reproductive age, a broad strategy that nevertheless hinged on notions of personal responsibility and individualized risk prevention.[109] Historian Al-Gailani makes the connection between the year the 1991 study was published and the formal announcement in the United Kingdom that "preconception care" would comprise a key component of maternity care services.[110] The construction of folic acid as a "risk-reducing drug" facilitated the advancement of clinical discussions around care for women before pregnancy, and efforts to promote pre-pregnancy care and pre-conceptional vitamin supplementation were "mutually reinforcing."[111]

In 1993, the lead author of the MRC study, Dr. Nicholas Wald, wrote the following:

> The critical timing of folic acid supplementation is not known but it is likely to be immediately before and during embryonic neural tube defect closure, that is, by four weeks from the date of conception or about six weeks from the first day of a pregnant woman's last menstrual period. There is necessarily uncertainty over when a woman will become pregnant, and she may seek medical attention only some weeks after her first missed menstrual period, which would be too late for folic acid supplementation to be effective. The general advice to women, therefore, must be to take folic acid supplementation from the time they decide to try to become pregnant. Failing that, the use of supplements immediately after a woman suspects she is pregnant is likely to confer a benefit in a proportion of cases, but to what extent is unknown.[112]

Wald's quote made clear that, even though the timing of the effect was inconclusive, the period around conception was deemed newly important. After a heated scientific debate over the timing effect and the safe amount of dosage, the U.S. Food and Drug Administration (FDA) issued a final rule in 1996 to fortify the nation's grain and cereal supply with folic acid.[113] Compliance with this rule became mandatory in 1998.[114] One government administration official remarked that the FDA rule would presume "all women are pregnant unless proven otherwise."[115] Pregnancy no longer presented the burden of proof for women to face recommendations for a healthy pregnancy, and thus prenatal care represented an intervention too late for preventing one of the most common congenital birth defects. The zero trimester was beginning to take shape.

Notably, the research attention to folic acid emerged alongside greater attention to the role of embryonic and fetal development in the medical literature. Obstetric ultrasound had become a common method for seeing the fetus.[116] Medical innovation and technology thus made it easier to regard the fetus as a patient and focus more than ever on fetal health and well-being, but there was also rising visibility of the *embryo* soon after conception.[117] By the 1980s, studies expanded previous research from the earlier part of the century[118] to show that the nervous system in human embryos is in formation by approximately twenty days post-ovulation.[119] This science matters for the present discussion because the 1980s witnessed a growing research agenda on pre-pregnancy interventions—such as folic acid—that might positively impact very early embryonic development and thus offset the risk of birth defects.

Moreover, the research on folic acid supplementation and NTDs coincided with the emergence in the 1980s of the "fetal origins hypothesis," also known as the "Barker hypothesis." The fetal origins hypothesis, as presented by Dr. David J. P. Barker, postulated that there are long-term effects of fetal exposures, effects that might not become visible until much later in life.[120] Indeed, immediate effects of fetal exposures—and realization that the placenta was permeable—were already apparent through birth defect disasters such as that experienced with the drug thalidomide and with the German measles epidemic of the mid-twentieth century.[121] The Barker hypothesis, though, renewed concerns about life-course health as setting the stage for healthy reproduction and also bolstered an epigenetic idea; that is, Barker's notion suggested that some underlying mechanism "programs" risk susceptibility, in which portions of the epigenome are switched on or off during the fetal period.[122]

The foundation for a renewed medical focus on early embryonic development—and on interventions that would enhance the environment of that development—set the context for the renewed rise of "pre-pregnancy" thinking in the world of obstetrics and maternal and child health in the late twentieth century. Reproductive medicine had a new golden tool for reducing risk.

EXPANDING AND DEBATING REPRODUCTIVE
SURVEILLANCE

As mentioned throughout this chapter, many contemporary maternal and child health professionals assert that pre-pregnancy care began in 1980 with an article on "prepregnancy clinics" in the *British Medical Journal* by Geoffrey Chamberlain. Chamberlain's clinic initially was set up in 1978 as a place for women to learn about risks to their health and the health of their future baby. The clinic identified maternal risks (e.g., previous pregnancy complications or current conditions, such as epilepsy) and fetal risks (e.g., previous multiple births or recurrent abortions). Chamberlain argued that an obstetrician should run a pre-pregnancy clinic.[123] Letters in response to Chamberlain's article questioned the novelty of his pre-pregnancy clinic idea: such a clinic had been set up in Australia in 1979[124]; women in a London practice had reportedly requested pre-pregnancy "check-ups" since 1969.[125]

Soon after, in 1981, the *British Medical Journal* ran an editorial on "preconception clinics." It argued that the question concerning whether obstetric care should begin *before conception* should be given "careful consideration," despite the fact that some physicians deem this only a "philosophical" question.[126] It would be a chance for obstetricians to counsel women with chronic conditions, the editorial argued. This piece also cited the recent "suggestions" by Smithells and colleagues in the *Lancet* about early evidence regarding folic acid and neural tube defects. The *BMJ* editorial evinced temporal reasoning in promoting pre-conception care as a new extension of the management of pre-pregnant women: "At present women usually present to the obstetrician for the first time with symptoms suggesting the fetus is *already jeopardized*. . . ."[127] Physicians during this time might have been dismayed at their lack of control over the early prenatal period, when embryos are growing rapidly, when women are not yet seeking care, and when the fetus is "already jeopardized." Some letters in response to this editorial jumped on the bandwagon, adding occupational hazards and alcohol as potential exposures women should avoid in the pre-conception period to avoid harm to future embryos.[128] One physician argued that a pre-pregnancy clinic would be a great place to warn women about alcohol reduction and the impact on pregnancy, buttressing his contention with the mention that Americans and their surgeon general have already included "all women who are contemplating pregnancy" to stop drinking.[129] Another physician argued that a pre-conception visit would "improve the obstetrician's ability to manage the pregnancy."[130]

It is clear from this discussion in the medical literature that pre-pregnancy care could increase the surveillance capacity of obstetricians over their patients. These early obstetrical proponents argued that there are specific embryological risks which might not be well understood but for which there is a need for physician oversight. The *BMJ* editorial, for instance, made a bold claim—one that would continue throughout subsequent medical literature on pre-pregnancy health: that potential damage to the fetus is done during the time when the pregnancy is unsupervised. If risks of adverse outcomes are in place during this early embryonic period, a discussion about the necessity of prenatal care was obviated to some commentators at the time. Prenatal care would continue to serve as *treatment*, not prevention.

By 1982, there was growing interest in health care around the time of conception and its impact on the reduction of birth defects and infant well-being.[131] One study found that a clinic helped management of diabetes in pregnant women "particularly at the time of conception and throughout the first trimester."[132] These advances were mostly attributed to the greater monitoring capability that physicians had over pregnant women's conditions and behaviors around the time conception occurred, not care in the months prior to pregnancy.

Some clinicians linked emergent ideas about pre-pregnancy care to the changes in women's social roles. For instance, one article in a nursing journal started off by noting that more women than ever were entering the labor force: "Additionally, today's working woman is increasingly interested in her health—before, during, and after pregnancy. Questions about preconceptional health needs are common . . . [a woman's] general health and state of nutrition at conception set the stage for health throughout the pregnancy. Her infant is affected by all of her past and present health habits. Preconception nutrition counseling can have a direct positive bearing on the outcome of pregnancy."[133] This statement was built on the growing recognition in nutrition studies of folic acid and fetal origins that implicated women's health status around the period of conception as of paramount importance to the woman's health and the health of her future fetus, but it was also concerned with changes in women's social status.

Going forward, the medical literature on pre-pregnancy health envisioned a new form of pregnancy risk management in the clinical setting. In the mid-1980s, additional calls percolated for obstetrics to expand formally to the pre-pregnancy period. One physician wrote that pre-conception and antenatal clinics must be the "foci of attention" for primary prevention, especially regarding alcohol risks to the fetus: "Most girls and pregnant women are aware of the danger of drugs to the unborn child in early pregnancy but unfortunately, they may not realize that alcohol is the most common drug to which they are likely to be exposed."[134] Mentions of risks to the "unborn child" were common in this literature. In the *American Journal of Obstetrics and Gynecology*, physicians specializing in reproductive medicine argued that the 1980s should be the decade of expansion into pre-pregnancy and post-conception counseling.[135] This reasoning for expanding obstetrical reach included the professional landscape that had accompanied the new trend of treating the fetus as patient. It was their obligation, these physicians argued, to monitor and assist mothers from the moment of conception, which meant also to prime women for pre-pregnancy awareness of clinical need. Yet, just as physicians questioned the efficacy of prenatal care in its early beginnings, physicians from all specialties were questioning the need for pre-pregnancy care and expanded reproductive surveillance.

In 1985, a short piece in the *Lancet* questioned whether "dragging" birth and pregnancy backward is really what women want.[136] As the *Lancet* column suggested, bringing conception into the medical realm appeared to be a new case of medicalization of the reproductive process, one that was perhaps unwelcome to women themselves. Formalizing a pre-pregnancy care service required pulling the period around conception into the medical realm and under medical supervision. This reality pointed to logistical questions about where women's health services would be located and who would get reimbursed for so-called pre-pregnancy services.

Letters to the editor in U.K. medical journals pointed to the professional hurdles that clinicians would have to endure with this new approach, arguing that patient demand is very low for pre-pregnancy health care.[137] One expert decried the use of pre-pregnancy clinics despite any potential gains by stating that "given the likely benefits and the investment required, particularly when there are other considerable demands on GPs' [general practitioners'] time, it is impossible to justify the existence of specific pre-conception clinics."[138]

Another physician wrote that there is nothing inherently novel in the idea of health before pregnancy and that making it a clinical event would cause unnecessary headache:

> Finally, I hope women are not really going to be encouraged to attend a booking clinic as soon as pregnancy is suspected. If all the women a couple of weeks late for a period were to see a consultant obstetrician before having at least a pregnancy test, which the GP can most appropriately arrange, then I am sure there would be little time left for gleaning a greater understanding of the causes of spontaneous abortions and fetal anomalies.[139]

Here, even in a comment supposedly targeting the pre-pregnancy health literature, the focus is on early pregnancy.[140] Physicians were not really debating pre-pregnancy health; they were debating how best to monitor the period of early pregnancy. This physician also clearly thought that obstetricians were encroaching on his jurisdiction as a general practitioner; he argued that he already offered general health care for women prior to pregnancy.[141]

Two more physicians published an article in *The Practitioner* (U.K.) that essentially "reminded" the medical establishment that general practitioners, at least in the United Kingdom, already do pre-pregnancy care. They conceded that it makes sense for obstetrics because they already have the antenatal clinics, but "since counseling before conception is conducted by general practitioners, specialists, and nurses, there is no need to set up preconception care clinics."[142] Notably, the U.K. health-care system is arranged quite differently than that of the United States. The U.K. literature highlighted debates about the necessity of a pre-pregnancy service when women already see obstetrician-gynecologists or general practitioners for preventive services. In the United States, prominent pre-pregnancy health researchers argued for various institutional placements, from how the obstetrician should expand his or her work, to how the pediatrician should intervene in the inter-conception period,[143] to how family practitioners can "do" obstetrical work.[144]

MOVING TOWARD THE ZERO TRIMESTER

The term "preconception care" in the United States was promoted most vigorously in the second half of the 1980s by two clinicians at the University of North Carolina—Chapel Hill, Robert Cefalo and Merry-K. Moos. They would become well-known as the earliest proponents of expanding obstetrics to include pre-pregnancy care. Moos and Cefalo's 1987 article in the *American Journal of Perinatology* argued that "recent medical research and a review of embryology suggest that interventions directed toward the preconceptional period may be a legitimate and overdue focus for the practice of modern obstetrics."[145]

Of course, Moos and Cefalo's writing emerged concurrently with ongoing questions about the efficacy of prenatal care. In the 1980s, maternal and child health experts and policy makers doubled down on prenatal care, hoping that expanding its services would improve population health measures such as infant and maternal morbidity and mortality. Yet, the 1980s emerged as a decade in which there was increased anxiety over the seeming inefficacy of prenatal care to combat problems of adverse birth outcomes, especially premature birth and infant mortality.[146] Progress on health markers had stalled, and the United States lagged further behind other developed countries on measures of infant and maternal mortality.[147] It was becoming clear that prenatal care was not doing what obstetricians had promised it would do in the United States. Maternal and child health experts began to call roundly for a "new perspective on prenatal care."[148] By 1980, some physicians saw the relationship between prenatal care and infant mortality as "restricted."[149] Other physicians and scientists called the evidence for prenatal care "flimsy."[150] While prenatal care was promoted as *the* answer to infant mortality in the early part of the twentieth century,[151] statistics revealed that twentieth-century improvements in maternal mortality and infant mortality predated the universal utilization of clinical prenatal care.[152] As Moos has written more recently, "For nearly 100 years, our nation's basic approach for preventing reproductive casualties—early and continuing prenatal care—has remained largely unchanged. The evidence that traditional prenatal care is equal to contemporary prevention needs is scant, yet inordinate amounts of public and personal resources are expended on the tradition."[153] Care during the three trimesters was not doing much good when it came to prevention of adverse birth outcomes.

Most of the experts I spoke with in the course of my research still believed prenatal care to be an important component of pregnancy care at the individual level; yet, they had all become acutely aware of what had been discussed elsewhere in health care literature as the "myth" of prenatal care.[154] One epidemiologist I interviewed explained it to me this way: "Stop thinking that you can fix everything during that little window of time known as pregnancy. That is ridiculous." Some major organizations made statements that reflect this sentiment. The Institute of Medicine's landmark 1985 report on U.S. women and pregnancy, *Preventing Low Birthweight*, highlighted pre-pregnancy conditions related to a woman's health that might impact the high rates of low birthweight in the United States. The report claimed that "healthy pregnancies begin before conception" and emphasized pre-pregnancy risk identification.[155] The report also expanded beyond obstetrical care and suggested that pre-pregnancy care be offered by obstetrician-gynecologists, nurses, primary care providers, pediatricians, and through family planning clinics. The report specified neither technical nor scientific evidence for a comprehensive pre-pregnancy care program; rather, it simply proffered that it might be time to shift the clinical focal point of risk assessments to pre-pregnancy to at least try for better birth outcomes.

The U.S. Public Health Service, in its 1989 publication, *Caring for our Future: The Content of Prenatal Care*, devoted an entire chapter to pre-pregnancy care and getting women's behaviors and conditions under clinical control prior to pregnancy.[156] Around the same time, the *British Medical Journal* reviewed legislation in the U.K. House of Commons related to maternity services in the country:

> The committee began at the beginning, or even earlier, by lending a sympathetic ear to arguments for systematic preconceptional care. It provided a platform for research suggesting that the health of both parents for 12 weeks before conception definitely affects the outcome of pregnancy. This was supported by medical witnesses only to the extent that preconceptional care should begin early, for example, by warning girls that smoking might not only cause cancer at 60 but might also harm their babies at 20. What was undisputed, the committee was told, was a connection between low birth

weight and poor nutrition during pregnancy, and the need for proper trials "so as to convince the medical profession." . . . Would a trial benefit the scientific community or the nation's mothers?[157]

This depiction allowed the "suggestion" that health prior to conception "definitely" affects pregnancy outcomes. The statement also revealed tension between the state of the science (discussed in more depth in Chapter 4) and potential interventions on women, using the morally-tinged phrase "nation's mothers."[158]

Cefalo and Moos also published the first clinical text on preconception health services in 1988, entitled *Preconceptional Health Promotion: A Practical Guide*.[159] The second edition was published within the span of a decade, entitled *Preconceptional Health Care: A Practical Guide*.[160] The pre-pregnancy framework moved between these editions from focusing predominately on health promotion to focusing on operationalizing the idea within clinical care. In 1990, physicians Brian Jack and Larry Culpepper wrote in the *Journal of the American Medical Association* of the growing attention to reproductive risks prior to conception, and they thoughtfully noted that pre-conception services might not be possible due to the inadequate access to care in many communities. They also argued that pre-conception care would "empower women to make informed decisions about childbearing," while also reducing adverse birth outcomes.[161]

In the 1990s, the Department of Health and Human Services's "family planning objectives" included expanding the proportion of primary care clinicians who provide pre-conception services to at least 60%.[162] Pre-conception care was also listed in *Healthy People 2000* as a maternal and infant health priority, solidifying the position of the idea in both family planning and maternal health.[163] In 1995, the American College of Obstetricians and Gynecologists (ACOG) released its first "technical bulletin" on pre-pregnancy care. The document's initial paragraph included this statement:

Some patients are unaware that their medical conditions, medications, occupational exposures, or social practices may have consequences in the earliest weeks of pregnancy. Because organogenesis begins around 17 days after fertilization, steps to provide the ideal environment for the developing conceptus are most likely to be effective if they precede the traditional initiation of prenatal care. Awareness of this fact has resulted in recent emphasis on preconceptional counseling.[164]

Despite using equivocal phrasing such as "may have" and "around," the risk facing the embryo was presented as fact. In addressing the growing literature around pre-pregnancy health and health care, ACOG attempted to make a statement about its recognition of the pre-pregnancy care model and to add legitimacy to growing worries about risks posed in early pregnancy.

Research in the 1990s also closely examined the association between family planning and pre-pregnancy health. Those women who intended their pregnancies were found to be more likely to avoid risky behaviors prior to pregnancy,[165] thus experts argued for pre-pregnancy care programs to combat unintended pregnancies.[166] Some of these articles deployed rhetoric indicating that women should plan their conception so as to have their pregnancies under better control, and thus extend the period of pregnancy. These types of articles highlighted unintended pregnancies as the social problem *du jour*. Popular books began to seize on the extended pregnancy idea as well, such as in one advice book titled *The Twelve-Month Pregnancy*.[167] At the turn of the twenty-first century, the March of Dimes declared prenatal care as occuring too late, and unintended pregnancies were deemed the prime target for new interventions.[168] Moreover, maternal and child health experts were calling attention to persistent racial disparities in birth outcomes and advocating a new life-course approach to maternal health care, of which pre-pregnancy care was typically mentioned as a crucial piece.[169]

Focus thus increasingly was placed on pregnancy intentions and family planning as factors that exacerbate poor outcomes in maternal and child health in America, underscoring the idea that pregnancies could be and should be deliberate and optimized. Pregnancy intentions, in particular, were ever more discussed as a social problem, especially in as much as the rise of effective contraception intersected with discussions of pregnancy optimization. Over the course of the twentieth century, there was a clear shift away from assessing specific risks in risky pregnancies toward the goal of optimizing every pregnancy. Not only did the end of the twentieth century witness a high rate of adverse birth outcomes and high rates of unintended pregnancies, but also apparent was a demographic shift wherein women were waiting until later in life to have children and were having fewer children overall—expanding their time in the so-called prepregnant period.

In 2006, the CDC marshaled the trend in the medical literature toward rethinking prenatal care, and accumulated the pressing problems of the day into a *Morbidity and Mortality Weekly Report* (*MMWR*), titled "Recommendations to Improve Preconception Health and Health Care—United States." *MMWR* releases are often called the "voice of CDC" and serve as "the agency's primary vehicle for scientific publication of timely, reliable, authoritative, accurate, objective, and useful public health information and recommendations."[170] The recommendations outlined in this *MMWR* publication linked issues of health and health care[171] and were devised as "a strategic plan to improve preconception health through clinical care, individual behavior change, community-based public health programs, and social marketing campaigns to change consumer knowledge and attitudes and practices."[172] That is, the report promoted the amelioration of social problems along with the clinical optimization of pregnancies. The authors of the *MMWR* document argued that progress on health measures—such as preterm birth and low birthweight—in the United States had "slowed, in part, because of inconsistent delivery and implementations of interventions before pregnancy."[173] Indeed, they averred that "for certain conditions, opportunities for preventive interventions occur only before conception."[174]

The report included attention to interventions on the individual level, but it also went into detail about how pre-pregnancy care would benefit population health. For example, it called for health insurance expansion for low-income women and argued that "affordability of care is a major concern for multiple women, and improved access to prenatal care is needed"; moreover, "approximately 17 million women do not have health insurance, and they are more likely to postpone or forgo care."[175] Pre-pregnancy care had been rebranded as the universal "fix" to social problems in addition to multifactorial causes of adverse pregnancy and birth outcomes in the United States. With the concurrent launching of the CDC's "Preconception Care Health and Health Care Initiative," pre-pregnancy health and health care suddenly became a major public-health concern in the United States.

POPULATION HEALTH AND SOCIAL ORDER

This chapter examined the historical underpinnings of medical knowledge regarding pre-pregnancy health and health care. Apparent from this analysis is that the pre-pregnancy health concentration in the medical literature has been driven not only by medical curiosity but also by perennial social concerns. Societies are invariably interested in the production of their future generations. As such, both social and medical thought have long converged on questions of what to do about mitigating reproductive risk and how to think about what kinds of interventions should be pursued and when.

In the nineteenth century, young girls were urged to take care of their health for maintaining their prospective maternity status. In the late nineteenth to early twentieth centuries, pre-pregnancy health status was the focus of syphilis campaigns, urging proper lifestyle among men and women and promoting "responsible" marriage. Pre-pregnancy health was a target in eugenics campaigns in the early twentieth century as well, urging individuals to think about their reproductive futures for the betterment of the race and the nation. For much of the second half of the twentieth century, as the focus on healthy pregnancies turned more and more toward the womb and prenatal care, however, pre-pregnancy health discourse dimmed in focus.

The knowledge construction around the pre-pregnancy care approach was often overshadowed by prenatal care, but then matured at an exponential pace as the influence of prenatal care dwindled over time. Increasingly, focus on improving birth outcomes shifted away from specific, identifiable risks during a pregnancy and more towards the woman and her lifestyle behaviors both before and during a pregnancy, coming full circle to the nineteenth-century notion that women's lives and lifestyles are important because women are the nation's future mothers. Reproductive surveillance became less about a specific period—nine months—or a specific body part—the womb—but rather about the whole of a woman's reproductive body and life span.

Pre-pregnancy health care discussions have waxed and waned over time in the medical literature. As mentioned at the beginning of the chapter, many experts cite Chamberlain's article in 1980 on pre-pregnancy clinics as a critical juncture in the contemporary clinical focus on pre-pregnancy health. Chamberlain's article was hardly the beginning, but it may be used as an effective pivot point to see how he relied on prior medical literature that focused on understanding risks as they arose *during pregnancies.* Chamberlain was seeking to achieve better results in the *next* pregnancy for a particular woman who had experienced a prior adverse outcome.[176] Exceedingly, after this period of Chamberlain's "pre-pregnancy clinics," the literature began to target *every woman* of childbearing age—not just women with a confirmed track record of poor reproductive results—and thus began the shift toward optimizing every pregnancy that is characteristic of today's pre-pregnancy care framework.

Medical knowledge about pre-pregnancy risk factors did not change drastically over time so much as it kept expanding to encompass more and more of a woman's life course as well as additional social and medical problems. Although pre-pregnancy interventions had previously emerged as magic-bullet approaches, especially with the folic-acid supplement studies, nothing of the scale of the CDC's work to define pre-pregnancy care and outline its broad range of possibilities had been attempted before the publication of an *MMWR* on the topic in 2006. The CDC's influential report codified new directions in the medical literature toward optimizing every pregnancy, reducing unintended pregnancies, and situating individual responsibility for reproductive risk. It additionally called directly for social change in health care provision and services for all women and, especially, for low-income women. As pre-pregnancy health discourse emerged in a prominent way in the twenty-first century with the CDC's involvement, pre-pregnancy care was promoted as a fix for both medical and social problems of the time: persistent adverse birth outcomes, high rates of unintended pregnancies, and inadequate access to preventive medical care.

The next two chapters turn to examining the work of producing and deploying the CDC's influential 2006 report—a document that would take pre-pregnancy care discussions out of the elite world of medical publications and catapult them into the public consciousness.

3 Anticipating Risky Bodies

MAKING SENSE OF FUTURE REPRODUCTIVE RISK

Modern medicine and public health can be understood as grand attempts to tame the future, to contain risk, to exert control where control is not fully possible.[1] And yet, to harness future reproductive risk—as pre-pregnancy care attempts to do—is to confront the reigning presence of uncertainty: we cannot foresee all risks to future pregnancies, and we cannot be sure that addressing specific risks in women's bodies and behaviors now will result in better outcomes later. That is to say, where the future is concerned, gaps in knowledge are conspicuous. Sociologists and historians of medicine have powerfully shown how medical and scientific knowledge does not always hinge on stark facts but rather is often shaped and filled by cultural dynamics.[2] The role of cultural undercurrents—for example, general understandings about women's reproductive responsibilities—in the navigation of uncertainty might be even more pronounced when critical consequences are at stake—such as the health of babies.[3]

As Chapter 2 detailed, pre-pregnancy health and health care were mentioned throughout the twentieth-century medical literature, but such references were largely as an afterthought to prenatal care. Increasingly, though, as prenatal care was failing to improve maternal and child health outcomes in a number of ways, experts began to subscribe to the idea that a woman enters pregnancy in poor health, thus positioning the locus of pregnancy health risk no longer in the pregnant woman but in the pre-pregnant woman. Crucially, these ideas essentially were conjecture; research articles did not exist to explain a direct evidence base for pre-pregnancy care. Yet, as the twentieth century came to a close, major agencies and organizations such as the Institute of Medicine, the U.S. Public Health Service, and the American College of Obstetricians and Gynecologists lent credibility to the idea of pre-pregnancy care by arguing simply that paying attention to it *might* prove to be a sensible way to think about improving reproductive outcomes. A rhetoric of guesswork indeed was typical in pre-pregnancy care publications (as it is in much of medicine and health discourse). In one of the first papers to recommend pre-pregnancy care in a major medical journal, Dr. Brian W. Jack and Dr. Larry Culpepper wrote in *JAMA* in 1990 that it is "intuitively advantageous" to pursue knowledge about risk factors prior to pregnancy.[4] A March of Dimes nursing module from the 1990s explained that "no studies have established the absolute effectiveness of this method of prevention" but that "it ultimately makes more sense to intervene before a pregnancy begins than after conception."[5] How did medical and cultural sensibilities about pre-pregnancy care take hold amid gulfs of knowledge? How did the idea of pre-pregnancy care become intuitive and coherent in the eyes of medical experts and public-health officials?

Drawing on the interviews I conducted with a "core set" of experts involved in the CDC's initiative for pre-conception health and health care,[6] this chapter delves into the meaning-making behind the pre-pregnancy care model at the turn of the twenty-first century to explore whether and to what extent experts relied on an evidence base to craft the pre-pregnancy care model. The official word in the medical literature or from CDC publications, as examined in Chapter 2, is one representation of a knowledge shift in thinking about risk. But how did the experts charged with drafting pre-pregnancy care policy positions and recommendations actually think and talk about pre-pregnancy risk and responsibility? How did the experts assigned with developing a pre-pregnancy care model perceive the need for this new direction? How did they come to an understanding about what causes poor birth outcomes, and how did they decide where to situate risk and levy reproductive responsibility? What explains the widespread belief in the importance of pre-pregnancy care among health professionals today?

This chapter scrutinizes how the need to focus on reducing health risks to pregnancies *before pregnancy* became "common sense" among health professionals and policy makers—even when the evidence to support this assumption was considered equivocal. It shows how evolving knowledge and strong cultural ideas about women's responsibility to take care of their bodies for future children worked together to make pre-pregnancy care an intuitive idea among practitioners.

What emerged in my interviews with the experts was a consistent theme of uncertainty regarding evidence for pre-pregnancy care, and experts employed specific strategies for addressing such uncertainty. Discussions of knowledge gaps were generally coupled with the belief that women enter pregnancy in a risky state and that women pose risks to fragile embryos, largely through lack of pregnancy planning and unhealthy lifestyles. Experts often presented as "fact" the scientific foundations of pre-pregnancy care, but deeper engagement with the words and beliefs expressed in the interviews revealed that these "facts" were inflected with social and cultural assumptions, inescapably laden with moral valuations and collective ideals about the locus of reproductive risk. Understandings about evidence were steeped in scientific findings and social assumptions about reproductive risk that were not *directly* related to the pre-pregnant period but that were proposed as tangentially germane, all the while drawing on the cultural potency of tropes about responsible motherhood. Moreover, an entrenched sense that more medical intervention is beneficial drove the development of the idea for a new "fix" for reproductive-health problems. The first section below details the construction of the select group of pre-pregnancy care experts. Then follows an analysis of how, in pursuing an elusive ideal of perfect babies, experts relied on cultural assumptions about reproduction—namely, women's ties to reproductive responsibility—to craft a new "common sense" about reproductive risk.

CONVENING THE EXPERTS

In June 2005, the CDC collaborated with the March of Dimes to assemble the first National Summit on Preconception Care. Concurrently, the CDC organized an expert Select Panel on Preconception Care, in which top researchers were charged with developing a comprehensive strategy for a pre-conception health and health care initiative, culminating in the publication of the influential 2006 *Morbidity and Mortality Weekly Report (MMWR)* document.

The CDC in June 2006 next convened a set of expert workgroups, and then created another select panel of experts in 2007. There was some overlap in participants among these meetings. The individuals I interviewed were involved in one or both of the select panels and some were part of the expert workgroup meeting. The experts I interviewed thus closely flank the publication of the *MMWR*, and they offered specific, though retrospective, accounts of this critical juncture moment in the history of the pre-pregnancy model as well as their general views on its basis and trajectory.[7]

The pool of experts can be grouped into two categories in terms of their background in pre-pregnancy health work prior to the CDC's meetings: "established experts," those who had conducted research specifically on pre-pregnancy health or health care prior to the CDC's initiative, and "new arrivers," those who heard about pre-pregnancy care for the first time when they were invited to be part of the CDC's initiative. Respondents who had published in the topic area prior to the CDC initiative cited the work by Cefalo and Moos at the University of North Carolina in the 1980s— mentioned in Chapter 2—as the first information they had read about pre-pregnancy health or health care. Experts specifically mentioned the clinical text, *Preconceptional Health Promotion*,[8] and Moos and Cefalo's 1987 article in the *American Journal of Perinatology*[9] as formative moments in the beginning of pre-pregnancy health discussions. Even if a respondent had not read the work by Cefalo and Moos, he or she still referenced them as the first advocates of pre-pregnancy care. In fact, several participants referred to Moos as the "grandmother" of pre-pregnancy care.[10]

The majority of the experts I spoke with fell into the group of "new arrivers" who were working on issues peripherally related to pre-pregnancy health. Before the CDC's initiative, many of the new arrivers had never heard the term "pre-conception care" or "pre-pregnancy care." This unfamiliarity changed with the work of Dr. Hani Atrash, who was then at the CDC's National Center on Birth Defects and Developmental Disabilities. Atrash, a trained obstetrician and public-health expert who specialized in birth defects and global infant and maternal mortality, spearheaded the pre-conception care initiative at CDC.[11] Despite all the earlier research and advocacy about pre-pregnancy care in the medical literature in the 1980s and 1990s, most experts I interviewed deemed Atrash *the* pre-pregnancy advocate—the one who initiated the national conversation. Alongside Atrash in this endeavor sat Kay Johnson, a renowned maternal and child health policy expert who had worked with the March of Dimes Birth Defects Foundation in the past and was hired by the CDC as a consultant to coordinate the pre-pregnancy health and health care initiative. One public health expert I interviewed reflected a common sentiment by referring to Atrash and Johnson as the "champions" of the pre-pregnancy care model. This text returns to a discussion of Atrash's central role again in Chapter 4, turning attention to the reproductive justice elements of pre-pregnancy care. It is worth noting here, however, that Atrash and CDC leadership brought pre-pregnancy care to the foreground of many experts' thinking. The following is a typical response received after asking an expert whether pre-conception care was a novel notion: "I guess I certainly understood that things that you do prior to pregnancy affected birth outcomes, and certainly I knew about folic acid. So some of the interventions I knew about. But as a package, I wouldn't say that I had heard of it [prior to the CDC meetings]" [public-health researcher].

The CDC's initiative "packaged" pre-conception care as a host of interventions, including genetic screening, recommendations about cessation of alcohol and non-essential prescription drugs, and recommendations about folic acid supplementation, among many other things. Although almost all of the experts had engaged in research or health promotion on a specific topic (e.g., fetal alcohol syndrome, diabetes, folic acid), very few had thought of pre-pregnancy care as a bundle of clinical services and health promotion messages. When asked to recall the first time reading or hearing about pre-conception care, the following response was emblematic of a "new arriver":

> It might have been when the workgroup that the CDC had helped to organize was putting forth the guidelines and recommendations related to preconception care. That might have been around the time that I heard about it, initially, in a formal way. Of course, pre-conception health or pre-conception care has always been a part of the work that I've done. So the topic was never new, because we were always speaking about how to get women who are not

pregnant, and possibly not even planning pregnancy, to start thinking about things like taking a multivitamin and making sure they have enough folic acid. [public-health researcher]

This expert had long worked on folic acid promotion for non-pregnant women and, like many other respondents, believed that pre-pregnancy *health* was important—this was not a new idea—but had never thought of pre-pregnancy *care* as a formal concept until the CDC convened the expert panel. Thus, the *model*—focused as it was on *self-care* through health promotion endeavors that target health behavior change, as well as on *health-care*—was deemed an innovative idea.

At the same time, the "established experts" found it intriguing—or, as one clinician put it, "amusing"—that many in the meetings thought that the CDC had just come up with the idea. Across the board, however, respondents reported that they were aware of the supposed importance of pre-pregnancy health before the CDC's initiative. All individuals I interviewed agreed that the health promotion and clinical focus of pre-pregnancy care did not emerge on a widespread scale until the CDC's involvement. The CDC, as a federal and influential organization, was instrumental in shaping ideas about pre-pregnancy care. Its leaders in maternal and reproductive health were key in stimulating the process of molding cultural ideas into accepted medical knowledge.

The experts were brought together to discuss the package of strategies concerning pre-pregnancy health care and health promotion practices. That is, they were summoned not to issue a recommendation about a particular intervention that might or might not be established within the medical literature, but rather to define and deploy a new holistic health risk approach—a suite of recommendations about health behavior, health promotion, and health care. To undertake this significant task, the evidence for such a broad and universal recommendation had to be parsed. By 2006, when the CDC published the *MMWR*, many advances had been made regarding the evidence of specific pre-pregnancy interventions, such as folic acid or diabetes control. But deep uncertainty remained—not only when it came to specific, individual-level interventions but most especially for the bundle of care interventions and for advocating pre-pregnancy care for all women of reproductive age in America. The 2006

MMWR publication recommending pre-conception health and health care acknowledged as much. Although the report defined the evidence for specific pre-pregnancy interventions as "definitive," it also explained that "limited evidence is available to determine effective methods for delivery of preconception care and preconception health."[12] Neither the medical literature nor experts themselves were all that convinced that such a care model was based in evidence—or that it needed to be.

EXPLAINING THE EVIDENCE FOR PRE-PREGNANCY CARE: IT'S "EVOLVING"

In light of the model's vagueness, pre-pregnancy care emerged as part of a new risk algorithm that had unformed evidence to fortify it. When uncertainty appeared, the cultural potency of "responsible motherhood" often filled knowledge gaps. A standard question in my interviews called upon the experts to describe or explain the evidence behind pre-pregnancy care. Almost everyone I interviewed mentioned folic acid supplementation and diabetes control as the best examples of pre-pregnancy care that are "evidence-based" and as "the precursor to what we're doing today" [public-health researcher]. One expert explained that folic acid is "the cornerstone of more concrete intervention" because "you can give a pill to women and see the effects" [physician], reminiscent of a "magic bullet" approach to health.[13] As discussed in previous chapters, folic acid's efficacy is in very *early pregnancy*. It is recommended prior to pregnancy so as to cover the early pregnancy period, when a woman might not yet know of her pregnancy. Nonetheless, experts consistently cited folic acid as the best example of a *pre-pregnancy* intervention, discussing it rhetorically as if pre-pregnancy folic acid intake directly and uniformly *causes* better birth outcomes, in the way that penicillin causes a bacterial infection to disappear. Pre-pregnancy care recommendations such as taking folic acid resonate with pervasive cultural understandings that "responsible mothers" should reduce all possible risks to children or future children.[14]

In my exchanges with experts, almost all described the evidence for pre-pregnancy care interventions as weak or tentative. For example, pre-pregnancy research was described as "emergent science" [general

practitioner] and an "evolving area" [public-health policy expert]. As one
respondent said, "to be quite frank, there's not a lot of studies yet that have
shown that pre-conception and inter-conceptional care will have an
impact on birth outcomes, yet," indicating that "we still have a lot of work
to do to test our theories in the realm of practice" [public-health
researcher]. That is, this theory of risk reduction was not yet considered
verified; and, to this end, experts were engaged in knowledge work around
future risk, initiating a policy program based on theoretical assumptions
about what interventions might interrupt the likelihood of future risk.
Some thought the lack of evidence for the pre-pregnancy care framework
presented a significant problem: "Yeah, I think we need to build the evidence. I think it can be very damaging to be pushing some general agenda
that doesn't have evidence. And I think [this lack of evidence] will under-
mine the whole process [of pre-pregnancy care advocacy]" [obstetrician].
One expert gave the following explanation when I asked what evidence
existed for pre-conception interventions:

> Well, I think that the challenge [for pre-pregnancy care] is that there's evidence
> for a lot of the individual sort of component interventions. There's not much in
> terms of the package and so sort of translating the individual intervention—
> that evidence—into a package level or, you know, sort of higher order factor
> model, if you will, is undetermined. And that's really, I think, the big challenge
> and the big question. . . . [For] some [components] . . . there's less evidence and
> it's not as compelling . . . but in other places, it is. . . . So, you know, the answer
> is there is and there isn't. [epidemiologist]

The statement that "there is and there isn't" evidence encapsulated so
much of the uncertainty and tension in experts' accounts of their involvement in the CDC's pre-conception health and health care initiative.
Experts believed that interventions prior to pregnancy impacted pregnancy outcomes, but became stymied in conversation by the seeming
dearth of "hard" science to back up their claim of the need for a shift in
how to think about reproductive risk. As one respondent said, "in terms of
how to deliver [pre-pregnancy care] comprehensively and in an effective
way, that's where the evidence is really lacking" [scientist].

Whereas the experts I spoke with did worry that a dearth of
evidence could undercut the model, many were also quick to explain that

pre-pregnancy care simply "makes sense." The following quote from an expert reflects a typical response:

> I really think [pre-pregnancy care is based on] the passion that people have, and they believe in the science. Pre-conception care is evidence based. Like I said ... just look at folic acid. You look at some of the other things—[like] women not using alcohol—there are things that we know that are evidence based. And then there's a passion also for public health and the whole thing about public health is we want to keep going upstream with public health. We were able to get prenatal [care] but then pre-conception is the next frontier after prenatal [care]. And [pre-pregnancy care is] primary prevention and that's what we want in public health is primary prevention. And it makes sense: a healthy woman and a healthy family. And [so] the things that we can attend to or attenuate prior to conception, we should try to. [scientist]

This scientist toggled back and forth between "evidence" and "passion," between "science" and "sense," highlighting a cultural trope that a healthy woman will make a healthy family. Accordingly, then, practicing "primary" prevention would be undertaking medical surveillance of women's bodies in the pre-pregnancy phase to try to reduce risk, foreshadowing a theme of distinctly *clinical* interventions that the text returns to later in this chapter.

Many experts expressed their conviction that pre-pregnancy care was worth pursuing by using terminology such as "logical," "obviously," "no brainer," and—as the quote above references—"sense" to explain their belief in it despite the proclaimed dearth of "evidence." For all the academic literature and discourse on life course health and singular pre-pregnancy interventions (e.g., folic acid, diabetes control), the experts consistently expressed that there is startlingly little evidence base for a pre-pregnancy care *model*. Nevertheless, this acknowledged lack of evidence for a broad-based package of recommendations did not emerge as a reason to withhold support. For those charged with defining and promoting the pre-pregnancy care model, the intuitiveness of the idea overshadowed any deficits of science.

Indeed, it was not clear that scientific evidence even could be harnessed to support pre-pregnancy care. The following interview quote is from an expert explaining how obtaining conclusive science would be difficult with pre-pregnancy care due to multiple complications for conducting "good" research in this area:

Now, the problem as I see it right now [with pre-pregnancy care evidence] is that I don't know that ethically you can do a randomized control trial. First of all, I'm not even sure that's the proper methodology to answer the question. . . . You want babies that weigh more? Do you want fewer birth defects? Do you want babies that have less, you know, obesity by the age of five? What is it that you're looking for because the outcome of pre-conception care is the quality and in some ways the quantity, which is affected by the quality of that life. Okay? And the mother's life. Well, that's such a huge multifaceted variable, I don't know that you can ever ask a discrete cause and effect question and come up with an answer for it. So I think that right now we have an increasing amount of data. I think people that are waiting and saying, "Well, until you do your randomized trial and have the single bullet answer," the response is, "This isn't the kind of a topic or question that lends itself to a single bullet." [obstetrician]

This obstetrician denied that randomized trials make sense for pre-pregnancy care because the question that needs answering is unclear. Randomized controlled trials are usually conducted to assess a *single* intervention.[15] The interventions to address preterm births might be very different from interventions that address overweight babies (e.g., from maternal diabetes). So, with this very complicated risk picture in mind, in which the "magic bullet" answer is not a single intervention but a more diffuse model of risk-reduction, experts generally returned to the supposition that it "makes sense" that healthy women will produce healthy babies. The following quote from another expert reveals that "common sense" might be all that is necessary to advance medical agendas:

A lot of it is just based on common sense. Like, there's data to show that controlling your blood sugar prevents birth defects if you're a diabetic. There's data to show the benefits of folic acid to prevent certain kinds of structural birth defects. But, there are almost no prospective randomized trials to look at other aspects of health care that, you know—does losing weight make a difference? I mean, it would make sense that it would, but there really aren't scientific studies out there showing it. In terms of behavioral changes, there are almost no data on it. So a lot of what we advise is just based on common sense. . . . But I'm not sure—for a lot of these behavioral changes [such as smoking cessation]—I'm not sure we absolutely need to have quality scientific evidence to support the advice we're giving. I mean, I do think there's a lot to be said for common sense. [obstetrician]

As reflected in this quote, a theme emerged that too much focus on "science" and "evidence" is misplaced. Another respondent explained to me that we should not focus too much on the "science" of pre-pregnancy care because all science "is biased, based on the participation of volunteers . . . there's flaws all over science; there's flaws all over the place" [epidemiologist]. Experts at times wondered aloud if a scientific underpinning was even necessary for the pre-pregnancy care framework. In the world of evidence-based medicine, is "common sense" enough to create new medical agendas? In seeming affirmation, some experts sometimes brushed aside my question about the evidence base for pre-pregnancy care. Others protested that we have never had good evidence for prenatal care, so why would we need good science for pre-pregnancy care? Such formulations could have significant consequences for the surveillance of women's bodies: approaches that are based on cultural and moral assumptions can move in many directions given the prevailing attitudes of the time regarding women's reproductive responsibilities. As prenatal care has institutionalized the surveillance of pregnant women, even while being a somewhat delinquent care model for addressing pressing population health problems, so pre-pregnancy care has the potential to concretize a new kind of widespread surveillance of the reproductive body.

One expert reminded me that "science does not change policy" [scientist]. Experts instead often relied on extra-scientific values. Another respondent said, for instance, that pre-pregnancy care is the "morally" right thing to do, a different argument of course than basing the model on something like clear facts: "Medicine hardly ever—and clinical care hardly ever—is all that linked to good evidence. For all of the evidence-based medicine in this country, much of what we do has no evidence base whatsoever. [For example,] prenatal care to me is primary care for women during pregnancy. It's good care; I'm glad she's getting it. I think it's morally a good thing to do. I think it actually has some positive benefits, just not in dramatically changing birth outcomes of the babies" [scientist].

Ballantyne himself—the "founder" of prenatal care in the early twentieth century, as described in Chapter 2—hedged about the potential efficacy of prevention programs targeting even *pregnant* women. In 1902, he wrote, "Here, on the very threshold of the subject, we meet with a check; for, when we come to consider it, we realize that about the physiology of pregnancy . . . our knowledge is very imperfect. . . . As a matter of fact, the profession does not understand the physiological changes of pregnancy."[16] Ballantyne suggested profound obstetric uncertainty when recalling his first case at the maternity hospital in which he diagnosed, before birth, a "malformed infant," when in fact the woman gave birth easily to healthy twins—"Such was the almost ludicrous termination of our first attempt to forecast the future of antenatal affairs," he wrote.[17] More than a century later, with the rise of the pre-pregnancy care framework, maternal and child health experts continue to grapple with uncertainty when it comes to understanding reproductive risk and interventions that might mitigate it.

There is no doubt that scientists and practitioners usually face uncertainty in their work and must manage the credibility and influence of their efforts,[18] and obstetricians and maternal and child health experts—as expressed by Ballantyne in another era—have long managed the challenge that comes with not understanding the etiology of birth outcomes. Amid uncertainties, the "fix" to health problems was portrayed in the contemporary CDC initiative as one based on "common sense"—one that pivoted on discussions of evidence that were not exactly pertinent for pre-pregnancy care but were closely related, as is shown in the following section. Additionally, this "common sense" was explained through making a case about women's risky behaviors and women's reproductive responsibilities in the contemporary reproductive-health landscape.

EXPLAINING THE MEDICAL PROBLEM: WOMEN ENGAGE IN RISKY BEHAVIOR WHEN "THE BABY'S ALREADY FORMED"

As mentioned in previous chapters, many specific pre-pregnancy behavioral habits do not have a clear connection to fetal outcomes. Although it is generally good for an individual's health to quit smoking, for example, and it would make sense to most people to stop smoking if planning a pregnancy, there is a tenuous relationship between smoking cigarettes at any time in the period prior to pregnancy and adverse effects on a future pregnancy or fetus. Smoking *during* pregnancy is related to ill effects, and research increasingly shows that smoking around the time of conception is, too. If a woman has not smoked for years, however, would her previous life choices come back to haunt her chances for a healthy pregnancy? Of course, it makes reasonable sense for physicians to advise women to stop smoking before getting pregnant. It is scientifically misleading, however, to claim a direct effect between a pre-pregnancy health behavior during a woman's reproductive years and a pregnancy outcome. What dominated experts' rationale for the pre-pregnancy care framework was the observation that women usually do not—or cannot—quit behaviors such as smoking in the earliest part of pregnancy, and experts depicted rapid embryonic development during such a phase of reproductive unawareness as of utmost importance in determining pregnancy outcomes. That is, even though experts did not offer *causal* connections between pre-pregnancy behaviors and future fetal damage, they did speak at length about other kinds of clear evidence related to pregnancy—that of embryonic organ development, biochemical risks posed to pregnancy by chronic conditions, and familiar research on the general medical effects of smoking or drinking. In formulating a justification for the pre-pregnancy care model, the experts made an ostensibly logical association: advice for a healthy pregnancy must also apply to pre-pregnancy health. Significantly, this is a hypothesized association, yet the pre-pregnancy care model is treated as "common sense" with scientific backing. Experts explained the need for "logical" pre-pregnancy care by invoking allied and already-recognized scientific research. In this rationalizing approach emerges a blending of indirect scientific reasoning with prevailing cultural suppositions about women's behavioral ties to reproductive outcomes.

Experts' discussions about engaging in fewer risky behaviors did not just apply to women planning to have kids imminently. In an interview, one respondent explained that "when you talk to adolescent girls at school about their health you also send a message that if you're healthy and don't engage in risky behavior like smoking . . . and if you choose to become pregnant in the future that [behavior] will help you get a better pregnancy outcome" [obstetrician]. Again, such advice is likely sound for a woman planning a pregnancy. Yet, a young person listening could interpret this statement as telling her that any and all unhealthy behavior she engages in today poses risk for any future pregnancies she may have.

A typical way that closely-related science was brought to bear on discussions about how pre-pregnancy care "makes sense" was the inclusion of data about embryogenesis and organogenesis, or the biological development of embryos and their organs. The experts often reflected common statements found in the medical literature and obstetrics textbooks when discussing how much development takes place before a woman ever presents for a prenatal care visit, such as in the following description provided to me in an interview:

> You know, from an embryologic standpoint, that all the major organ systems are either complete, or in the process of being developed, by the time the average woman gets in for her first prenatal visit. So the whole story of pre-conception care is that if we're waiting for prenatal care to be the answer, then we've missed eighty percent of the organ development. And anything that a woman does, unfortunately either through intentional or unintentional exposure to teratogens or toxins, or anything—the harm has already been done. So I think [pre-pregnancy care is] really trying to widen the lens, and back up, and see [pre-pregnancy care as] more of a lifecycle issue than actually around a specific event of a pregnancy. [general practitioner]

Indeed, much fetal development begins well before a woman usually realizes she is pregnant. Typically, women are not aware of their pregnancy until about eight to ten weeks of gestation. During the first eight weeks of development—which marks the embryonic period—the neural tube, lips, eyes, ears, genitals, and other organs begin to form.[19] Similar to the quote above, in which the expert explained how "the harm has already been done" by the time a woman enters prenatal care, another expert also cited facts about organogenesis and said "the action is over" by the time a woman presents at a prenatal care visit:

> I mean, I don't know that prenatal care isn't a good thing. Nobody can do the randomized trial of taking half of the women and giving them prenatal care, and half not. *I think that probably a lot of what's going on, in terms of what the outcome of the pregnancy is going to be, is sealed by the time the woman realizes she's pregnant.* You know, if there's going to be a birth defect, the organs have already started forming before she realizes she's pregnant. If she's going to develop a condition like pre-eclampsia, [this] has to do with placentation, and placentation is already well underway by the time she realizes she's pregnant. So if she's going to [have an] impact on something like pre-eclampsia or growth restriction, those things have already happened. So [the issue] may be if you're going to have someone quit smoking,

it's better to have her quit before she gets pregnant. *A lot of it is sealed by the time the woman gets pregnant.* So if you're going to have her change her health habits, or optimize her health, and have it result in an impact on her pregnancy, it's got to be done before she actually gets pregnant. *Because a lot of the action is over by the time she gets into prenatal care.* [obstetrician] [emphasis added.]

The temporal blurriness that appears with much pre-pregnancy care discussions is emphasized in this quote. The expert here stated that fetal outcomes are probably already "sealed" *by the time* a woman realizes she is pregnant. Later in the quote, the expert stated that the future is likely already "sealed" *before* the woman ever gets pregnant, and then finished by saying that "a lot of the action" (meaning fetal development) is over by the time the woman enters prenatal care—another temporal marker. Whether the critical period is prior to pregnancy or after conception is unclear; no matter, the best course of action, according to this expert—and to the pre-pregnancy care model—is to have women optimizing their health prior to getting pregnant. By so doing, all the relevant time periods are covered. Every risk is anticipated; every risk-mitigating behavior enhanced.

To many experts, the rise of the pre-pregnancy care framework served as an important counterpoint to what they perceived as a lack of medical and lay consideration of the early embryonic phase of gestation. As the quote above suggests, regarding fetal development, "a lot of it is sealed" by the time the physician sees a pregnant woman. This sentiment mattered to the experts I interviewed because of the potential harmful effects occurring in the interim. Take the following quote as an example:

[Prenatal care is] clearly not helping. It's not helping because even though women are getting prenatal care, the birth outcomes aren't improved. I mean, from a medical perspective, if you just look at that clinical component: let's say a woman has diabetes, and she doesn't know that before she gets pregnant, [and] her blood sugar is out of control. By the time she comes in to the clinic, at seven, eight, nine weeks, that baby's major organ systems are already formed. She has high blood sugar? There's nothing you can do. That baby is already going to have possible—you know, that sugar can have teratogenic effects on that fetus. [public-health researcher]

This expert, as did many, referred to the embryo as a "baby," suggesting a clear focus on how risks to embryos *now* might turn into *future* risk to babies, and highlighted how the "baby" is damaged well before a clinician ever sees a pregnant woman. Another expert told me, "the baby's already formed by the eighth week of gestation . . . you need the right environment for implantation [or] that's how you get birth defects" [general practitioner]. The sentiment in this quote was typical, and it suggested a direct cause of birth defects: imperfect attention to self-care and health care, whether the woman has a chronic condition or whether her lifestyle is considered unhealthy. Suggesting that "the baby's already formed" during this phase of development obviates discussions about the remaining developmental time in a fetus' or infant's life.

Birth defects have many causes—some demonstrably unknown or unknowable—but considerations in reproductive-risk discussions often are centered on the need for women to change their lifestyle behaviors to correct perceived imperfections. Operating here is the current cultural emphasis on perfection in reproduction, a focus that elides discussions about anything that detracts from the supposed goal of flawless reproduction. Scholars have noted this cultural shift toward creating perfect babies, either through an intense focus on women's behaviors or through the use of science to avoid reproductive chance.[20] Experts I spoke with argued that many of the pressing problems they see facing maternal and child health today are because of "behavioral manifestations" that impede optimal reproduction—things over which, as one expert put it, "people have control if they want to have control: smoking, drinking, risky behavior—that sort of thing" [obstetrician]. That is, many of the interviews revealed an abiding belief among experts that women should change their lifestyle and behaviors, and that without such changes women are putting their future pregnancies in precarious positions. To be sure, many of the individuals I interviewed acknowledged how difficult it is to change behavior. Still, the answer was often simply that women should stop engaging in risky behaviors in the first place. For example, experts worried about unchecked chronic conditions, such as with diabetic and obese women, as the following excerpt revealed:

> So, it's not only getting the environment so that the uterus isn't all sugared up and you've got an awful hostile environment for implantation which you've got to [treat]—glycosylated proteins take a while to turn over, so that's why you want some time to get rid of, you know, the environment to

[make] all the proteins normal, so you need a normal blood sugar. And once your sugar's normal, if we have given permission to get pregnant—a lot of women ask that question: "When will you give me permission to try?" Because there are a lot of women who are in terrible glucose control and they're planning pregnancy. We say to them, "You know, for heaven's sake, you only have one or two or three times to be a mother. Let's just plan." [general practitioner]

In this quote, women who are diabetic host "an awful hostile environment for implantation." Furthermore, this statement intimates that it is the clinician who is positioned to give "permission to get pregnant." This comment also taps into cultural attitudes toward precious pregnancies and normative notions of childbearing—as women "only have one or two or three times to be a mother" in contemporary society. In referencing risks to embryos, fetuses, and babies, many of the experts referred to women's gestating role and one of women's most salient social roles: mother. Highlighting the master status of motherhood outlined a strategy used by many experts to underscore the importance of pre-pregnancy care. As in the quote above, experts also consistently mentioned chronic diseases—usually diabetes and obesity—that characterize the current moment in U.S. health-care burden. According to experts, women's generally flippant attitude about their reproductive lives and women's high rates of chronic disease put pregnancies in peril.

Of course, clinicians have not always thought that embryos and fetuses were so vulnerable, or that women's bodies were so risky. In fact, for much of the twentieth century, medical experts thought of the fetus as a "perfect parasite"—taking exactly what it needed for optimal growth, no matter the woman's behavior or context.[21] Historian Angela Creager has discussed how the permeability of the placenta was not even recognized until the 1950s.[22] Except for nineteenth-century ideas about maternal impressions, the fact that women's bodies might be inhospitable to fetuses across the board—and that fetuses are ultimately impressionable—is relatively new. As also briefly mentioned in Chapter 2, the scientific, medical, and cultural shifts that occurred in the second half of the twentieth century toward an understanding that the maternal environment could matter significantly for fetal development—along with the rising medical visibility of pregnancies (e.g., with the introduction of ultrasound technology) and the increasing sense that every pregnancy is precious, especially given that women have fewer pregnancies and children than ever before—led to the current moment in which embryos, in addition to fetuses, are highly valued. Thus, embryos today are perceived to be in jeopardy without women's proper prior awareness and control.[23]

Not every person I interviewed dwelled on the individual woman's body as a potentially hostile environment; several experts thoughtfully mentioned broader environmental forces that fostered a hostile reproductive context. One nursing expert said that it is necessary to look at the "most toxic elements" of one's environment, be it a woman's own "biochemical physiologic environment" or "her place" in the larger social and political environment, which inevitably interacts "along with her genetics." This expert went on to explain:

> And so that entire interplay—that is just vitally important to consider for each woman, and that's why to just start to look at it once pregnancy is already [established], and once there's been conception, and most likely two months, three months into it, is starting way, way behind. . . . And you can only hope that you're finding someone who has all of those kinds of things in balance, and not that the factors going on that are going to contribute negatively to the fetal development. But that's unusual. In fact, we could say it's almost impossible, but on the other hand, what is our goal here? Our goal is not to create some perfect environment, whether it [be] your internal or your external environment. Our goal is to mitigate what we can. To prepare for what we can and to balance out what we can, so that it's the best possible environment for that baby—for that fetus to grow in and those women to be supported. . . ." [nurse]

This respondent, as did others before, clearly advances the argument that women and physicians usually start off far behind when pregnant women present to care—that, indeed, embryonic and fetal development usually outpace the typical care time line. This expert, however, further clarified that it might be impossible to create a perfect uterine environment—that, instead, the goal is to try to "mitigate what we can" and provide the "best possible environment" for both baby and mother. According to experts, the only way to do this effectively—the only perceived way to try to ensure the optimization of reproduction and motherhood—was to improve pregnancy planning.

TALKING TO WOMEN ABOUT OPTIMIZING
REPRODUCTION: THEY "REALLY HAVE TO HAVE
A PLAN," BUT YOU "DON'T WANT TO SCARE THEM"

Within the medical literature on pre-pregnancy health and health care that was reviewed for this book, as well as in the interviews I conducted, there emerged both an implicit and explicit insistence that reproductive-aged women are always at risk of potential motherhood and should act accordingly. Many experts surmised that the reason that women are engaging in risky behaviors and posing potential risks to their embryos and fetuses is because they do not adequately plan their reproductive lives. As the following interview excerpt suggests, women should be reproductively mindful and "aware":

> Really [pre-pregnancy care is] just a broadened understanding of, you know, it's kind of that big picture thinking that's very hard for a lot of us: that the behavior we have today has an [impact] down the road . . . if you're sexually active and not using birth control then you're probably, even though you're not planning on it, you could get pregnant. So you have to have other behaviors that would support that pregnancy if it did occur. It's a very complex behavior [change] I'm looking for. . . . Awareness! [public-policy expert]

Similarly, in the following excerpted answer to an interview question about how women might think about pre-pregnancy care, an expert argued that all women need to be aware that they can get pregnant—that they are reproductive bodies:

> Hm. How would I like [women] to think about health behavior? Well, I guess I just think that it would be helpful if there was a general awareness about the impact of [women's] health during the pre-conception period, even if they're not considering getting pregnant [and] that they can get pregnant. You know, all of the statistics that half of pregnancies are unplanned is a big issue in pre-conception health. So, just an awareness of the fact that they are reproductively capable, and that they need to take certain steps, like taking their folic acid, and you know, all those things that we talk about! [scientist]

"Awareness" was promoted as the answer for pregnancy intention problems and adverse birth outcomes.[24] Pregnancy intentions, though, are very difficult to understand. Individuals' reproductive behaviors are incredibly complex, and researchers have spent years trying to figure out why women have pregnancies that are "mistimed" or "unwanted."[25] Although an expert focus on family planning might seem at best helpful and at worst innocuous, organizational and provider insistence on the critical importance of "planned parenthood" in reality might cover up sources of inequality in the ability to plan or intend a pregnancy.[26] Additionally, sociologist Emily Mann has shown how reproductive health providers sometimes push young women—especially those in minority groups—to attach themselves to normative notions of pregnancy planning through using contraception even if the young women do not indicate wanting to avoid a pregnancy.[27] There is a mismatch between providers' insistence on reproductive awareness and women's realities.

Some interviewees understood this incongruity. As one respondent eloquently put it, "I think that we should start with determining whether or not [intendedness is] a valued concept to the women we care for. Because if we're selling something that doesn't matter to [patients], we're spinning our wheels!" [clinician].

Yet, despite the known intricacies of pregnancy intentions, many prepregnancy health professionals evinced a generalized assessment that women should just plan their pregnancies—a viewpoint that largely stemmed from their day-to-day work, wherein they reported seeing women who are not using contraception and who have no reproductive plan. The same respondent who questioned the focus on intendedness above also explained a typical clinical exchange with pregnant women: "I would say, 'Were you using birth control?' and they would say, 'No.' And I would say, 'Were you hoping to become pregnant?' and they would say, 'No.' And then I would say, 'Okay, so help me understand this.'" As a clinician, this expert found it frustrating that women's intentions and behaviors did not match their reproductive reality and—as did other respondents—demonstrated disappointment in women, not men. Cultural and medical assumptions about gendered responsibility abound when it comes to pregnancy intentions—and women are charged with undertaking the measures that are required to make sure pregnancies are "planned."[28] There indeed emerged a gendered and cultural tint to the language used by the experts that reflected the extent to which providers and society hold women accountable for reproduction *and* reproductive outcomes.

There was also an underlying supposition among most interviewees that women *should* plan and that they *can* plan their pregnancies (i.e., have access to contraceptives, have influence over their partner). But there often was not overt recognition that women engaging in what were deemed very risky behaviors (e.g., smoking, illicit drugs) also are women who might be at risk in ways that make it harder for them to plan in the first place. So, while much discussion centered on controlling risks to fetal health in the early embryonic stage, a parallel concern emerged among the experts about controlling conception itself. That is, a critical justification for pre-pregnancy care among the experts centered on its ability to be a model that can address pregnancy intentions. Most respondents believed pre-pregnancy care to be primarily an issue of family planning, arguing that "an unwanted pregnancy is a high-risk pregnancy" [public-health researcher]. The following excerpt from my interview with a physician reflects health professionals' concerns about unplanned pregnancies: "A lot of women don't plan pregnancy, and when they find out they're pregnant, then they decide to get healthy, and it's often too late. That's not a good time to start a new exercise thing. And by the time you realize you're pregnant, a lot of the major organs, including the neural tube, have already formed. . . ." [obstetrician].

Dr. Hani Atrash evinced a similar concern when discussing why prenatal care is inadequate. He explained:

> Why isn't prenatal care enough? Simply because we know that most of those conditions that cause adverse pregnancy outcomes—whether it's obesity or smoking or HIV or whatever—you don't manage them and cure them and successfully change them overnight: it takes time. It takes months or years sometimes, you know. And the other thing is if the woman is using drugs or is not taking folic acid by the time she knows she's pregnant, it's too late. And the average woman enters prenatal care at eleven weeks. . . . Most of the fetal organs—actually all of the fetal organs—are formed by the eighth week, so there's going to be damage to the fetus because of a health condition or a medication or an environmental exposure. It will happen mostly before a woman shows up at a clinic to see her provider for prenatal care. Or if she has a health condition or a behavior that she needs to change, it will take time from the first visit—it's not easy to stop smoking and lose weight, you know. All those things take a long time to do. [interview]

Concerns about embryogenesis in this quote and others above were inextricably linked with concerns about family planning. Thus, concerns were not simply focused on strictly medical and scientific topics; interrelated were social concerns about family planning and women's lifestyles in the United States.[29] The pre-pregnancy care model's focus on planning was envisioned to improve reproductive awareness and, by extension, improve birth outcomes.[30]

After establishing the importance of pregnancy intentions in their framework of risk, experts then had to ponder what they might tell women. There is a policy prescription, but there is also the clinical one-on-one interaction between a clinician and a reproductive-aged woman. A fundamental message of pre-pregnancy care is that "women need to see their health professional before they get pregnant, so that they can . . . be in the best possible health before becoming pregnant" [public-health researcher]. Yet, some experts were sensitive to the fact that achieving optimal health prior to pregnancy often is unreasonable and, indeed, some worried that the messages might make women unduly anxious about their reproductive bodies, as did one respondent, who stated, "for example, with diabetes, that does increase your risk of birth defects, having uncontrolled diabetes. So I think educating women about that, really making sure that they have their diabetes really under control and maintain it under control before they get pregnant and during their pregnancy. And really giving these women accurate risk assessments. I mean you don't want to scare them so much that they think you're telling them, 'well you can't have kids because it's just going to turn out badly'" [scientist].

Experts were quick to note that they did not intend to "blame" or "scare" women. They also observed the whole model as an uphill battle in terms of changing women's behaviors. One interviewee, for instance, explained that it is difficult to tell women to stop drinking: "Most people are not able to achieve that level of [alcohol] abstinence. So, [we need to] access women prior to getting pregnant and if they are not able to quit some of these risk behaviors [then] help them to postpone pregnancy until that safer period is achieved. So that you don't have the birth of a child affected with alcohol exposure or tobacco exposure or drug exposure. So this is all a way to minimize the final burden from this window period, you know, the first three months" [physician].

In this quote and in others that mention alcohol, there is an absence of discussion of actual evidence regarding alcohol and birth defects. Research is clear that heavy, chronic drinking during pregnancy can produce adverse effects, in some cases even the condition recognized as fetal alcohol syndrome,[31] and yet the "safer period" is determined to be achieved through zero tolerance. Awareness of the zero trimester helps reduce a "final burden"—an unfortunate turn of phrase—to the fetus, according to this mindset. The recommendation to women is simply to "quit some of these risk behaviors." As one expert explained: "It's just a question of: do I get her before she's pregnant, and get her under good control, and reduce the risk of her having a poor pregnancy outcome? Or am I playing catch-up by getting her at twelve weeks, when her baby's birth defect may have already happened? But either way, I'm going to be taking care of her. So there's no threat to me going out of business" [obstetrician]. Some clinicians thus saw risk as inevitable; the bigger concern to many of the experts was at what point they would be able to intervene.

THE CLINICAL TURN IN MATERNAL AND CHILD HEALTH

A focus on pre-pregnancy *health* might simply continue an anachronistic social statement about how important it is for women to prepare themselves as the nation's future mothers, but the *care* part of the pre-pregnancy risk framework—as the offspring of prenatal care—situates prevention of adverse birth outcomes in a clinical setting. Maternal and child health as a field has moved away from broader social policy interventions toward individualized medical interventions to address child health and well-being.[32] It thus seemed natural to the experts I interviewed that, in the twenty-first century, more clinical intervention and more health education and behavior change among women is the answer to healthier reproduction for generations to come. These responses reflected similar statements in the medical literature. In one article, for example, about the need for a pre-pregnancy care model, entitled "The Time to Act," Dr. Hani Atrash and colleagues noted: "One of the reasons that progress in improving pregnancy outcomes has slowed down, and in some cases reversed direction, is that we have failed to intervene before pregnancy to detect, manage, modify, and control maternal behaviors, health conditions, and risk factors that contribute to adverse maternal and infant outcomes."[33]

The urgency in this sentence stems from the failure of prenatal care as medical intervention; yet, the answer calls for even more medical intervention, revealing medicalization as an entrenched approach to addressing health problems, as well as the continual search for "magic bullets" in pregnancy health. This focus on clinical interventions for pre-pregnant women in the name of pregnancy-related outcomes represents a case of expanded medical monitoring of the reproductive body.[34] In many ways, the surveillance and screening that pregnant women already undergo with prenatal care made it easier for the pre-pregnancy care initiative to promote similar clinical interventions for pre-pregnant women. Certain tests, like preconception genetic screening, are easy to add to the clinical encounter because it is already "part of the medical model" [scientist]. It is this rooted sense of medicalization that pulls the generalized female reproductive body into the domain of medicine and within the purview of public-health surveillance. Medicalization begets medicalization.

Physicians that I interviewed noted that they see a lot of women who are prescribed too many pharmaceuticals,[35] and experts positioned pre-pregnancy care and medical advice as a way of reducing women's reliance on unnecessary medications, as in the following quote:

> You know . . . particularly nowadays it's really, really frustrating the number of women who come in in their twenties and they're on a myriad of medications. They have a whole slew of medical problems. Most of them quite honestly because they're obese and now they're diabetic and now they're hypertensive and no one ever stops to say to them, as they're lecturing them about losing weight . . . it hasn't dawned on anybody yet that this is a young woman who doesn't have kids yet and she's probably going to end up getting pregnant. So she really ought to be told, "Oh, by the way, we're putting [you] on these medicines, but you shouldn't get pregnant on them," or, "Oh, by the way, here's the risk if you happen to . . . get pregnant, with your obesity or with your diabetes or with your hypertension." [obstetrician]

This doctor envisioned the clinical potential for reorienting the patient to be properly prepared for pregnancy. Such preparation, of course, represents another encounter the woman will have with clinical advice and monitoring. Moreover, this expert believed that women must "be told" that they are not healthy enough for pregnancy. Indeed, most respondents felt that women should think about how their current behaviors will impact a future pregnancy. Medical advice in this way can become a form of social control.[36] Conversely, it also envisions pre-pregnancy interventions as empowering women, as the same obstetrician explained: "But I think [pre-pregnancy care] just reminds women . . . [that] 'Yeah, I am supposed to plan this. I am supposed to exert my authority and control over my reproductive choices and decisions and events.'"

Some respondents, though, were uncomfortable with the overtly clinical focus of pre-pregnancy care. One expert explained that pre-pregnancy health interventions had always made sense, but that the CDC's *MMWR* recommendations took a biomedical course and positioned the initiative on a distinctly clinical turn, saying, "people can make choices outside of the medical paradigm. So I was a strong proponent of pre-conception *health*, and opponent of pre-conception *care*, just because of what I perceive as the exclusivity, the issues of access, and the issues of locus of control" [scientist]. When asked if the pre-conception framework is reductionist, another expert answered, "To the degree that it gets defined as what you can do clinically and medically for a woman in a doctor's office, yes. But if you think about it more broadly, you know, how can we improve social conditions for women and how can we improve their access to services—those medical services and personal services? How can we help them change their behaviors so as to improve their health? Then I think it can be conceived more broadly" [scientist].

Experts who were steeped in a public-health background rather than a clinical background were reluctant to see clinical surveillance of women as the answer for improved birth outcomes, believing instead that a spotlight must be shone on a woman's social environment, such as that indicated in the following quote:

> [Prenatal care is] too late! It's too little! I mean, I think it's important. But you know what? Getting the blood pressure and doing the urine during a pregnancy those things, to me, they are not really as important factors as getting the girls to finish high school! I mean, I just think some of those other determinants of going upstream will probably have more to do with what kind of birth outcome you have—behaviors, you know, like smoking.

I think prenatal care is still important, but it's just insufficient. It is insufficient and we've got to take a much broader view. [pediatrician]

Experts further questioned whom they might be leaving out of a medicalized pre-pregnancy agenda, in which clinicians could potentially use reproduction and reproductive capacity as the precursor to comprehensive care. Experts highlighted population groups with the potential to be ignored in the pre-pregnancy framework, including women with mental health problems, women with disabilities, and gay and lesbian individuals.

While there was recognition that a pre-pregnancy care model might not be reasonable, and in fact might scare women or be too much part of a "clinical turn," many experts still highlighted the need for women to understand that they should be "in tight control" [scientist] before pregnancy. Yet, waiting and striving for a "safer period" for pregnancy is hard to operationalize. When are all the risks covered? When is it "safe" for women to get pregnant? Experts perceived pre-pregnancy care as an effective way forward in part because it extended the window of reproductive surveillance over risky behaviors and fragile embryos. Their understanding was framed in terms of rapid organ development during a time when pregnancy often goes undetected. With pre-pregnancy care, both women and clinicians would ostensibly exhibit enhanced reproductive scrutiny and optimized maternity through better planning. Scientific facts about embryonic development and general health behaviors were culled to make the case for a new temporal definition of reproductive risk, one that would be monitored by the health profession. All of this work to develop a new "common sense" about pregnancy health hinged on underlying assumptions about women's ties to reproductive responsibility and individualized medical risk.

GENDER AND "COMMON SENSE" IN AN ERA OF ANTICIPATORY MEDICINE

Pre-pregnancy care is characterized by a clinical and social concern about *future risk*, not about a condition that is extant now, but about one that might pose risk in the future. A woman of reproductive age who is not

pregnant might not pose any serious risks to her future fetus. Yet, anticipating risk and hedging uncertainty are key components of contemporary
medicine,[37] with the distinct feature of treating otherwise healthy populations as if they are already potentially diseased.[38] This trend toward "risky
medicine," as historian Robert Aronowitz calls it, focuses on expanding
previous disease categories by situating an individual as "at risk" of future
disease. The idea of the rise of "risky medicine" is not exactly synonymous
with the concept of medicalization, which characterized some of the "clinical turn" in maternal and child health discussed above. Medicalization
scholarship, rather than focusing on the expansion of established disease
categories, has focused attention on how non-diseases become diseases[39]—
in the way that, say, "normal sadness" becomes treated as clinical depression[40]—and to how, more recently, the ways in which medicine has become
transformed by technological science and risk mitigation.[41] I would argue
that pre-pregnancy care as an anticipatory strategy[42] traverses all these
concerns.

First, pre-pregnancy care expands medical jurisdiction over a "non-
disease" in the sense that it brings an otherwise "normal" state—the reproductive years of a woman—under clinical supervision like never before. By
clinically defining a woman's non-pregnant body as potentially risky to
her future embryo, her future fetus, and her future child, reproduction is
indeed further medicalized—even if in an anticipatory way.[43] Because the
"pre-pregnancy state" has been identified as a potential risk factor, it car-
ries with it the social process of (bio)medicalizing a putative risk that
might or might not appear someday.

Second, it also can be seen as expanding a "disease" state. Although
pregnancy is a completely normal component of a woman's life course, it
often is considered a "disease" in cultural and policy parlance. By calling
the years of a woman's life in which she has childbearing potential the "pre-
pregnancy phase," clinicians and health experts have expanded a clinical
and "disease category," encroaching on women's otherwise healthy bodies.
If a woman of reproductive age is defined as pre-pregnant, she is potentially harboring a "disease"—that is, women are always "at risk" of pregnancy in the pre-pregnancy care framework. Furthermore, non-pregnant
women acting as if they are pre-pregnant—the idea behind the ethic of

anticipatory motherhood—is illustrative of the contemporary risky-medicine notion of the converged experience of risk and disease.[44]

Pre-pregnancy care as an anticipatory care strategy, then, highlights how medicine and public health today focus on preemptive clinical intervention and on future risk. It also is a bellwether for where this trend is further headed: toward preventive interventions in the name of the health of future generations.[45] That is, pre-pregnancy care is pronounced by its future-body generational focus. Much previous scholarship on risky medicine and (bio)medicalization concerns extant bodies. Pre-pregnancy care highlights anticipatory care for multiple temporal landscapes.

Such a move toward future risk to future bodies as something that is within the purview of non-pregnant women's health profile is possible in part because women are thought of as reproductive vessels by default. The interviews discussed in this chapter lay bare that the connection between women and reproduction remains insuperable. It is—perhaps surprisingly— through science rhetoric that the cultural assumptions about women and reproductive responsibility come to the fore. Experts drew on related medical science and cultural constructions to justify and legitimate the pre-pregnancy care model. By using scientific claims that seemed to resonate with pre-pregnancy "logic," the experts were engaged in a process of filling knowledge gaps by fitting evidence to cultural assumptions about women as bearers of a nation's health. The justification of this new care strategy by an expert coalition helped establish a new "common sense" that pregnancy health begins well before pregnancy. Women's bodies were defined as risky pre-pregnant bodies in need of medical supervision to intervene in the fragile embryonic phase.

"Culture works by making some ideas natural and others unthinkable."[46] Health research and discourse can remake what everyone regards as common sense[47]; or it can instantiate and perpetuate what everyone considers to be accepted knowledge. To the extent that there were gaps in certainty and in clarity about reproductive risks posed by "women of childbearing age," these gaps were filled with language of intuition and cultural logic—that it simply "makes sense" that women of reproductive age should lead a healthy lifestyle and seek medical care to reduce risk to future fetuses and babies. In the case of pre-pregnancy care, employing and solidifying cultural ideas about women's bodies and reproductive responsibility remade common sense around pregnancy health.

The experts I interviewed thus neutralized the uncertainty around the science of pre-pregnancy care interventions by explaining related science and then leaving the rest of the agenda to cultural logic, reifying the general medical and cultural assumption of a strong tie between women's behaviors and reproductive outcomes. My objective in discussing this prevailing logic of pre-pregnancy care is not to determine when medicine or public health should use "good science" and when it should not. In fact, as several experts eloquently explained, it is often unclear even what "good science" would look like in such a complicated and complex arena as reproductive outcomes. The noteworthy finding here is how much of this "logic" about future risk comes to be predicated on related medical science and existing medical and cultural protocols of governing pregnancy and women's bodies. If, as one expert told me, "a woman is a mother from the time of her own conception" [pediatrician], then powerful cultural and gendered assumptions about women's lives and motherhood are bound up in the ways that experts think about reproductive care and reproductive risk.

I have focused here on the extent to which certain types of common sense imbricate and infuse all action that gets pursued in the reproductive arena[48] and on the extent to which cultural dynamics shaped thinking about pathways to reduce risk to healthy pregnancies in the United States. Placing reproductive responsibility disproportionately on women is not atypical in medical discourse; however, it is the idea of future risk that animates the current pre-pregnancy care model and further entrenches retrograde ideas about women and reproduction. Why, in the early twenty-first century, did a diverse array of experts draw on and validate such seemingly essentialist ideas about women, maternity, and clinical interventions? It is to this question that Chapter 4 turns.

4 Whither Women's Health?

REPRODUCTIVE POLITICS AND THE LEGACY OF MATERNALISM

When talking about my research on pre-pregnancy care, people have often looked at me, bewildered, and asked, "Don't you just mean 'women's health'?" A definition of "pre-pregnancy care" might seem straightforward. It is anything but. Achievement of such a seemingly unmoored definition is difficult in America, where women's health services and health coverage have long been defined not along the lines of womanhood per se but rather along the lines of motherhood or potential motherhood. Discussions about improving pregnancy care and birth outcomes usually fall within the world of maternal and child health, a realm of public health and public policy that is aimed primarily at caring for pregnancies, mothers, and children. Alternatively, discussions about *women's health prior to pregnancy* are decidedly not in the world of maternal and child health. Yet pre-pregnancy care conflates women's health with maternal health. It does so by definition.

In 2006, when the CDC formally recommended that women of reproductive age seek care prior to pregnancy in the name of pregnancy health, the general health status of women of reproductive age was reframed as maternal in nature. In short, all of women's health during their reproductive years was categorized as maternal health. It was perhaps this most basic question of definitions and boundaries that precipitated the initial backlash to the CDC's report, in which popular and scholarly commentary decried how CDC experts were defining women in an essentialist fashion. To some degree, critics seemed puzzled as to why a non-pregnant woman would need to seek maternity care or engage in "healthy pregnancy practices," and critiques seemed to conclude that such pre-pregnancy care messages must be anti-feminist in nature insofar as they equate womanhood with a maternal role. Observers perhaps have wondered how it is that—in the twenty-first century—physicians and policy makers basically treat women like reproductive vessels, asking non-pregnant women to seek out pre-pregnancy care throughout their reproductive lives in order to be prepared for inevitable motherhood.

The experts involved in drafting and disseminating the CDC's report were taken aback by the unflattering public responses. As I learned in my conversations with those involved in the CDC's initiative, they depicted their work in part as righting failures in the way that reproductive health services in America are organized, discussed, and distributed. The women's health arena—in which policies and politics are largely delineated according to whether a woman is pregnant or is a mother—presents a significant hurdle for caring for a woman across her life course. To the experts, it was previous policy arrangements that were retrograde, not the 2006 report advocating pre-pregnancy care—a report that responsively aimed to establish a holistic view of women's health across reproductive life stages. Moreover, pre-pregnancy care is a model that promotes expanded access to health services for women whose needs are otherwise often ignored by policy makers, such as those of poor women, women of color, and women seeking family-planning services.[1] As such, advocates claimed, pre-pregnancy care could be understood as a matter of reproductive justice.

That the emergence of the CDC's pre-pregnancy care framework produced such opposing interpretations—on the one hand, the model is backward; on the other, it is progressive—and that it sparked such confusion, and at times vitriol, about the definitions and boundaries of women's health services, taps into a long-held political and ideological divide in the United States between reproductive health and maternal health. In fact, by advocating for pre-pregnancy care, the experts involved in the CDC's work were traversing some thorny ideological and political territory. By targeting the improvement of *reproductive health* through a *maternity care* lens, the pre-pregnancy care model was decidedly in a murky space.

As did Chapter 3, this chapter looks behind the official words of the CDC's 2006 influential report and attends to the intentions and motivations of those involved in the work of producing and/or deliberating the report. The official report produced a new public-health policy imperative, one that hastened subsequent state and federal initiatives to improve pre-pregnancy health and health care and, in this way, it was quite clear in its programmatic prescriptions. But examining only the words and recommendations of the report leaves open many questions about the impetuses behind it. This chapter specifically places the CDC's report in the political context of the time of its publication, during the Presidency of George W. Bush and before President Barack Obama's push for health care reform. This timing matters because much of the political backdrop of the experts' words focused on expanding health care access and circumventing contentious reproductive politics. This chapter reveals that much of the thinking surrounding the construction and deployment of pre-pregnancy care in theory was not designed to be essentialist toward women, as many critics have presumed, but rather was considered among experts to be a political-economic strategy that was aimed at occasioning a paradigmatic shift in public health and medicine toward focusing on women's life-course health and reproductive justice. That is to say, to make sense of the thrust of the CDC's report is to understand experts' concerns about how in America reproductive care and services have been set up into reproductive silos—delimited as they are by the boundaries of maternal and reproductive health politics.

This chapter returns to the present work's core set of interviews to understand how experts positioned pre-pregnancy care in the women's health care and policy arena. It shows how—due to the legacies of reproductive silos and ongoing reproductive policy divisions—the experts envisioned pre-pregnancy care as a bridging concept, something that could facilitate a convergence of divergent reproductive worlds and advance reproductive justice. Amid this discussion, I include a short review of the policy history that established the reality of reproductive silos in America. In the end, I argue that the policy strategy of maternalism—characterized by defining women's needs in terms of their maternal status—guided and smoothed this bridging work. I also consider how maternalism remains a guiding policy theory and cultural logic in health strategies—one that continues to permeate thinking about gendered reproductive responsibility and the implementation of reproductive strategies.

If the previous chapter underscored how reductionist ideas about women as pre-pregnant bodies continue to shape medical thinking, this chapter complicates this story as it focuses on how pre-pregnancy care experts have been intent on founding a fresh foothold for reproductive justice. Indeed, there are complex layers and dualities inherent in crafting reproductive agendas. Still, the cultural resonance of motherhood emerges as a common denominator in thinking both about medical intervention and about reproductive politics.

THE MORAL CAMPAIGN

The experts who agreed to participate in the CDC's initiative for pre-pregnancy care did so for a variety of reasons. Those I spoke with reported having a long-standing commitment to maternal and child health issues, whether through clinical or public health work. Most experts also cited an underlying interest in women's health more broadly. Many of the older female experts I interviewed reported that they became passionate about their field of work through being involved in the women's health movement of the 1970s.[2] Experts thus began working in the CDC's initiative because they were asked to do so, and because they thought it would positively impact women's health and birth outcomes in the United States.

One obstetrician reiterated that pre-pregnancy care disappeared in maternal and child health discussions during the 1990s until Hani Atrash "resurrected the whole thing." Atrash had served in CDC's Division of Reproductive Health (DRH) since the 1980s, where he was a steward of the Safe Motherhood movement—a global initiative that aimed to reduce maternal mortality around the world by emphasizing women's health "before, during, and after pregnancy." When Atrash moved from DRH to the National Center on Birth Defects and Developmental Disabilities at CDC, it was no wonder that he already knew the research on the "before pregnancy" component of women's health. He saw an opening for pre-conception care to link reproductive health (an area often concerned with, among other things, family planning, contraception, and abortion) and maternal health (an area often concerned with prenatal and postnatal care)—areas that were somewhat separated by CDC divisions.[3]

In short, Atrash envisioned pre-conception care as a potential avenue for advancing discussions about the neglected importance of the intersections and interactions between reproductive health and maternal health, including their relationship with birth outcomes, and Atrash expressed a moral responsibility to pursue this work. He recalled: "The first lecture I gave on preconception care, in September 2004, my first slide was 'Preconception care—why should we care?' I think my second slide was— 'Because it's illegal, immoral and unethical for us not to'" [interview].

Sociologist Howard Becker in 1963 wrote that "moral crusades have strong humanitarian overtones," noting that moral entrepreneurs typically come from the "upper levels of the social structure."[4] Dr. Atrash could be considered a moral entrepreneur, and his career has markers of such a definition. His work has been devoted to addressing maternal and infant mortality and morbidity, and he has worked on these issues domestically and globally. He was deliberate about how his affiliation with an elite organization like the CDC is advantageous because it confers much legitimacy, credibility, and moral responsibility to work toward humanitarian goals. In the following quote, Atrash explains how he worked to forge what needed to be done to get these issues some attention in a social climate that tended to not care very much about women's health:

> We have women's health programs; we have family planning programs. But we also know that our country suffers from being thirtieth in infant mortality among developed countries. We still have a very high maternal death rate with a huge racial disparity issue. There are issues that the country has accepted as priorities that we need to deal with: preterm delivery, birth defects. All those issues fall under the umbrella of improving pregnancy outcomes. So if you present [pre-pregnancy care] as an "improving pregnancy outcomes agenda," it's more likely to be successful. [interview]

What is important in this interview excerpt is that Dr. Atrash understood early on that the bifurcation between reproductive health and maternal and child health at the CDC and beyond was not bringing anyone closer to solving health problems. Pre-pregnancy care, he believed, married the fields of general women's health and pregnancy outcomes, thus positioning a more successful enterprise for helping women, mothers, and babies.

As becomes evident in this chapter, the pre-pregnancy care model eventually emerged as a "valence issue" for those involved in the CDC's work—situated in such a way so as to be immune from political contestation.[5] Atrash and other pre-pregnancy care leaders purposefully organized a group of scientists, medical experts, and public-health specialists to assemble an exclusive collective for the task of disseminating "new" claims[6] about risks posed to pregnancy outcomes, claims that would be persuasive both scientifically and rhetorically.[7] Those involved in the initiative thus served as scientific and biomedical entrepreneurs[8] for the purpose of a moral campaign for healthier babies in America.

Dr. Atrash was a key entrepreneur, a central facilitator in the emergence of the pre-pregnancy care framework in the twenty-first century, and his work emerged at a particular socio-historical juncture—one in which fetuses had much visibility, in which babies were dying at much too high a rate, in which women were spending more of their life course not pregnant, and in which medicine was increasingly anticipating risk—that rendered his ideas highly palatable. As influential as his work was and has been, it would be misleading to attribute the social change made to Atrash alone. He helped to bring together what sociologist Steven Epstein calls a "tacit coalition"[9]—a group that incorporates many individuals' expertise to pursue a particular agenda.

The expert collective convened at CDC headquarters included specialists in family medicine, nursing, pediatrics, obstetrics-gynecology, epidemiology, dentistry, midwifery, and public policy. Some of the invited experts worked at CDC but many did not, and they flew to Atlanta from all over the country. The initiative was not driven by any particular specialty. As much as pre-pregnancy health and health care emerged from the obstetrics literature in the twentieth century, it was not only obstetricians who were involved in the CDC's work. Clinicians from diverse specialties were called together to address adverse birth outcomes and reproductive health and to craft ideas under the same "rubric" of pre-conception care, despite whether their day-to-day work focused on family planning, maternal health, or fetal health.

In essentially "rediscovering" pre-conception care as a major public-health concern and priority for the CDC, Atrash—along with other leaders at CDC including Dr. Samuel F. Posner—revived the older literature on pre-pregnancy health, galvanized the growing literature on pre-pregnancy health risk factors, and set in motion a whole new wave of research and collaboration on the topic of pre-conception care, to bolster both the science and the policy impact of the pre-pregnancy care model. Through Atrash's passion and the work of the initiative's participants, pre-pregnancy care became identified as a moral imperative to care about women's health, broadly, and birth defects, specifically, at the same time. Suddenly, in the twenty-first century, pre-pregnancy care was considered by many to be the "new" and best way to refocus health care toward the moral and comprehensive treatment of women and babies.

As detailed in Chapter 3, despite the lack of a clear evidence base that pre-pregnancy care would reduce risk, it nevertheless was positioned not just as something that "made sense" medically but also as the "right" thing to do for women and babies in America—as the answer for advancing discussions about how to improve the health of women, mothers, and babies. Based on the interviews conducted, the sections that follow offer that there are two chief reasons why such discussions about improving maternal and child health have been stymied or elided in the past, leading up to the perceived political need for pre-pregnancy care among many health experts in the twenty-first century: the legacy of reproductive politics and enduring divisions in reproductive health services.

REPRODUCTIVE POLITICS AND
REPRODUCTIVE CODE WORK

To talk about anything prior to pregnancy is to get mired in the unique arrangement of contemporary reproductive politics. Take the aforementioned Safe Motherhood movement as an illustrative example. Facilitated in part by the United Nations Decade for Women (1976–1985), a renewed call began in the 1980s for women's health and safe motherhood as human rights.[10] Yet, this also was the time of the rise of the conservative right in the 1980s that produced a political climate geared toward elevating the status of the fetus and being particularly hostile to women, women's rights, and women's health.[11] Obstetrics and maternal and child health during the 1980s also was increasingly focusing on the fetus. As a result, maternal and child health scholars began to question the lack of focus on mothers and, especially, on maternal mortality.[12] Public health scholar Lorraine V. Klerman, in referring to increased focus on pre-pregnancy health and maternal mortality in the medical literature, wrote that, "these objectives bring the woman and her family back into the prenatal care picture, which for the last several decades has been dominated by the fetus/infant."[13]

It was in this context that the global movement for "Safe Motherhood" arose, stressing the problem of maternal mortality by focusing on *women's health* broadly.[14] The idea of "women's health," though, had become markedly entangled with abortion politics, and Carla AbouZahr of the World Health Organization wrote of this problem for Safe Motherhood: "Among anti-abortionists, safe motherhood was seen as the Trojan horse for the introduction of legal abortion. Funders interested in supporting safe motherhood programmes became wary and today certain donors cannot be approached for support to projects or programmes that include an abortion-related component."[15]

While it is remarkable that an effort to reduce preventable death was controversial, this likely did not go unnoticed by the experts defining pre-pregnancy care. They were keenly aware of how any reproductive agenda that includes non-pregnant women risks being aligned with general reproductive health services, which includes family planning, contraception, and abortion. And pre-pregnancy health experts have long noted that family planning services represent a key part of pre-pregnancy care.[16]

Many of those involved in the CDC's initiative agreed that pre-pregnancy health is simply "women's health," but the prickly hangover of reproductive politics explained the decision to stick with the label "pre-conception" or "pre-pregnancy." In fact, for many experts reproductive politics emerged as the reason as to why the pre-pregnancy care model was needed in the first place, as such politics had obstructed women's health care. One resplendent recounted such deliberations, saying, "There was really a lot of discussion about people wanting to frame [pre-pregnancy health] as a women's health issue, and there was a lot of discussion back saying, 'We can't, because this is a difficult topic.' And for years, women's health has been ignored, because when you talk about women's health, you're talking about reproductive rights, and therefore you're talking about abortions, and no one wants to touch that!" [public-health researcher].

When asked to define pre-pregnancy care, many experts explained that it is code for "women's health," often even preferring the term "women's health" to "pre-pregnancy health." Why, then, the question often arose in my interviews, is "pre-pregnancy care" not simply called a new "women's health model?" Again, the answer was simple: women's health contains reproductive health and thus includes abortion. By framing a women's health approach in terms of pregnancy, the focus could stay within the world of maternal health. Thus, "pre-pregnancy health" became a coded tactic to talk about reproductive health and life-course health.

In interviews, experts were clear to note that "reproductive health" and thus "women's health" tended to raise their political antennae because of the associations with family planning, contraception, and abortion. Another pre-pregnancy health expert expressed a longing to call her work "reproductive health" or "women's health," but lamented that "when people say reproductive health and women's health, it's, 'Oh, family planning, abortion'" [public-health researcher], thus undercutting her desires. An expert in the same field believed that pre-pregnancy health was a "women's health issue" but realized that, "[pre-pregnancy care] needed to be framed at the time as a maternal and child health issue. Because for some reason, when you talk about women's health, it's a harder sell, because that leads you down the path of reproductive rights, abortion, and so we really struggled during the conference, in writing these recommendations, even though we wanted to frame it as a women's health issue, to kind of stay away from that, because it's kind of a hot topic politically" [public-health researcher]. A physician also explained: "I prefer to call [pre-pregnancy care] what it is: women's health. Up until now we've had so many schisms [and when] we start talking about women's health, people immediately go to the pelvis and abortion issue, because that's a polarizing factor" [pediatrician].

The "embattled" reproductive history in the United States had, according to one interviewee, "reduced women's reproductive health in so many ways to a conversation about family planning and abortion" [public-policy expert]. More than one expert articulated the sentiment that "if reproductive health wasn't code for family planning, STDs, and abortion," they would have called the model "reproductive health." That is, the way that experts talked about reproductive silos and reproductive care was generally arrayed by abortion. Thus, the timing of the need to define a new model outside of the reproductive health world had political underpinnings.

The following quote reveals how some respondents thought of the political climate as paramount:

> Under the Clinton administration there had been a lot of women's health initiatives funded. And then when the Bush administration came in they did away with a lot of that, and [the Bush administration] didn't want to hear the term women's health, and they clearly didn't understand it. I mean, there were always some people in the policy world who hear the term "women's health" and they think you're talking about abortion. They think it's a code word, which drives me nuts but that's another story. So, I know that the movers and shakers in the CDC group did not want to frame it as women's health. I felt that was wrong, but I was one voice arguing for that . . . I mean I think the whole thing is about women but [the challenge is] how you frame it and how you try to sell it. [scientist]

This scientist specifically used the term "sell" to explain the strategic utility of the term "pre-conception care." One prominent leader of the initiative was adamant in our interview that the pre-pregnancy care model was *not* a product of a conservative political climate that was exceedingly hostile to reproductive rights. To be sure, as Chapter 2 reveals, pre-pregnancy health discussions have been around for some time, irrespective of political administration. Yet, by contrast, many of those I interviewed expressed a clear belief in the vein of the quote above—that pre-pregnancy care was a savvy strategy during a particular political moment. One respondent even called the term pre-conception care "bullshit," implying that it had no meaning except for political utility [public-policy expert]. This same expert urged me not to focus too much on the language but rather on what the model actually was trying to achieve: expanded health care access, life-course care, and improved reproductive health status and birth outcomes. Of course, language matters; how and why we come to label ideas or policy prescriptions in the ways that we do reveals underlying cultural assumptions and concerns of the times. The political context might help illuminate why—despite rumblings of pre-pregnancy health and health care in the literature for more than a century—pre-pregnancy care emerged with such vigor in the twenty-first century.

It became apparent in my interviews that, contrary to many outside critiques that have been leveled at pre-pregnancy care, those involved in defining and deploying the model believed that pre-pregnancy health was simply a strategic way to talk about women's health, as something that is "applicable whether or not a woman intends to get pregnant or wants to get pregnant"—and not as a "presumption that the woman wants to conceive eventually and [that] she's trying to be healthy prior to conception" [public-policy expert]. That is, expert accounts offered a narrative that emphasized how pre-pregnancy care was meant to improve women's health and their access to health services overall by encompassing *both* maternal care and reproductive care. Yet this task was not going to be easy, as the realms of maternal health and reproductive health have long been, for many intents and purposes, alienated from one another.

PREVENTING BABIES VERSUS SAFEGUARDING BABIES: REPRODUCTIVE SILOS IN AMERICA

In calling attention to the politically contentious nature of reproductive-health services, experts spoke about the fractious manner in which such services have been set up over time in the United States. The reproductive silos of maternity health services and family-planning services have made it difficult for anyone to think outside of boxes demarcated by whether or not a woman is pregnant.[17]

This section takes a short foray into the history of reproductive silos in America and of state interest in pregnant women, to help establish— beyond the sheer politics mentioned above—the more specific policy context through which to make sense of a new policy imperative of pre-pregnancy care. Some of the legislation mentioned in this section is touched upon briefly in Chapter 2 as part of the historical advent of prenatal care, but I revisit and reiterate some distinct pieces of this history here, as this background helps to explain the political legacy that informed the twenty-first century drive for pre-pregnancy care as well as how CDC experts envisioned the model as a reproductive-justice project.

There is an extensive history of state interest in the as-yet-conceived; the United States in particular has an established social policy undercurrent of focusing on women as future mothers. Maternalist politics pivot on defining women's needs in terms of their maternal status, and women and politicians have historically been very effective at mobilizing a collective ethos of maternalism. As Theda Skocpol's work so thoroughly details, numerous social benefits in the early 1900s were orchestrated by civic-minded and engaged American "clubwomen" leading a maternalist vision of state building. In the late nineteenth and early twentieth centuries, social and political arguments linked maternity and women's needs in order to expand state welfare services and health care access to women and children.[18] During the first two decades of the twentieth century, numerous labor protections and social regulations were legislated by states and by Congress to "help adult American women as mothers or as *potential mothers*."[19] For instance, the famed 1908 Brandeis Brief in *Muller v. Oregon* argued for restricting the number of hours women could work partly on the basis of their social status as future mothers. A woman's reproductive capacity historically often has established her standing as a woman.[20]

Using maternalist politics, women sought expanded assistance for not only themselves but for their children. In the first two decades of the twentieth century, many social problems such as child labor and infant milk hygiene came to the forefront of public discourse because of the social reform movement led by women.[21] One major maternalist success in the early twentieth century was the establishment of the Children's Bureau. First supported by President Theodore Roosevelt and then signed into law by President Taft in 1912, the Children's Bureau represented the first time the federal government recognized an express responsibility for safeguarding the health of the nation's children. The Children's Bureau was composed entirely of women and was headed by a woman, Julia Lathrop.[22] Lathrop kicked off the new organization by initiating studies of infant and maternal mortality—a vital task, as no national database on infant mortality previously existed, and there was no good sense of the demographics of how many babies were born or died each year. This work was the first to document the fact that the United States had a high infant mortality rate as compared to other developed nations. The Children's Bureau—highlighting infant mortality and the poor U.S. ranking on the international stage therein—in 1913 published a pamphlet, *Prenatal Care*, which spurred the idea that pregnancy should be considered a medical event.[23] Prior to this era, as mentioned in Chapter 2, only women with medical complications saw a physician during pregnancy or childbirth.

The Children's Bureau also promoted the successful passage of the first federal social welfare program that offered grants-in-aid to states through the Sheppard-Towner Maternity and Infancy Protection Act of 1921. This Act was designed to spread health information to mothers, and to provide funding for prenatal and postnatal clinics.[24] Because of Sheppard-Towner, public health information about pregnancy and infant care proliferated and spread across the states, even into small and rural towns. Before the 1920s, maternal and infant health programs and services did not exist in many of these areas, especially in southern and western parts of the United States.[25]

And so *maternal and child health* in the United States has its beginnings in (mostly white) women's advocacy and leadership in the early part of the twentieth century. Women were capitalizing on trends to protect children and to protect women as mothers or even as *potential* mothers. Women used maternalist strategies to have a voice in promoting health and civic engagement—that is, they used their status as mothers or future mothers, not necessarily as women, to make a case for their political and security needs. The newly enfranchised female electorate prompted politicians into action on maternal and child health issues.[26] Any social benefits for women in these legislative victories were achieved through emphasizing their maternal role in the nation's hierarchy.

The historical twist to this success was that the Sheppard-Towner Act did not last long. Rising opposition from the American Medical Association, and the Act's designation as an annually-renewed appropriation (as opposed to a permanent entitlement like Social Security), left it in a vulnerable political position,[27] and it lapsed in 1929. Historian Sheila Rothman has argued that the demise of Sheppard-Towner was a punctuated end to female-led expertise in preventive health services.[28] The fall of Sheppard-Towner, though, did not spell the end of defining women's health in terms of maternal and child health. The Act was defeated, but maternal and child health programs did get taken up again soon enough.

Many of the desires of advocates within the Children's Bureau were carried beyond the Sheppard-Towner period into the 1930s. President Franklin

Roosevelt signed Title V of the Social Security Act (SSA) into law on August 14, 1935, and included federal grants-in-aid to states for maternal and child health services as well as for child welfare services. A longtime director of the Maternal and Child Health Bureau (1977–1992), Vince Hutchins, noted that it was a crucial distinction that Title V was part of the SSA, because as part of this piece of legislation it was recognized that "it is the dependence of children and mothers, rather than different diseases or health conditions, that prompts special attention to them."[29] That is, maternal and child health, as its own separate realm, was defined categorically in social policy as a critical part of securing societal well-being, especially during the Depression Era. It remained a crucial measure for securing health care for low-income women throughout the twentieth century, but usually only applied to these women when they were pregnant—that is, when they were on the cusp of motherhood.[30]

Title V has undergone amendments over the decades, but it remains the only federal program dedicated to safeguarding and improving the health of all mothers and children in the United States. It is today bureaucratically buried within the Department of Health and Human Services, administered by the Maternal and Child Health Bureau.[31] This reality is quite different from the dominant and visible position that maternal and child health held within the Children's Bureau a century ago.[32] Still, however, Title V remains a major silo of women's health, a silo that tends to ideologically align itself more with babies, and by extension pregnant women and mothers, rather than with women's health more broadly.

Provision of government-funded health insurance also highlights the state interest in pregnant women over general women's health. Passed as part of the Social Security Act of 1965, the Medicaid program has since aimed to provide health insurance for people in poverty and other individuals who are eligible by virtue of population group category or income status. In the 1980s, the federal government required that pregnant women and infants with incomes up to 100% of the federal poverty level be eligible for Medicaid coverage.[33] Before President Obama's health-reform bill, Medicaid coverage was limited to certain categorical groups, such as pregnant women, mothers, individuals with disabilities, and children. As health policy expert Sara Rosenbaum has pointed out, prior to Obama's health reform these categorical requirements would have prevented a low-income single woman of reproductive age from getting health insurance,[34] unless that woman lived in a state that had a waiver to cover such services.[35] Again, it was women's status as mothers or as expectant mothers and not their status as women that afforded comprehensive care. With private insurance plans, as well, coverage has varied over time and by plan on the question of whether it is inclusive of all the moments of care in a woman's reproductive life span (e.g., prenatal care, childbirth, postnatal care, Pap smears, abortions, contraception).

These last few reproductive subject matters are cordoned off in a different silo when it comes to health programs and funds for services. While the maternal and child health silo and consistent care for pregnant women was being codified in the policy realm in the twentieth century, a parallel policy push emerged for *preventing and spacing babies*—for birth control and family planning in the United States. This history has already been thoroughly documented by numerous scholars,[36] but the following highlights a few critical junctures leading to the establishment of the reproductive health silo.

Margaret Sanger illegally opened the first birth control clinic in 1916, in Brooklyn, New York. Planned Parenthood of America was formally established in 1942 to distribute birth control and offer family-planning advice, aiding women in their desires to prevent and space pregnancies. The first federal grants to support family planning occurred under the Johnson Administration as part of the War on Poverty and linked population policies to both class and race.[37] In 1970, under President Nixon, family planning was solidified and bolstered by the passage of the Public Health Service Act. The Act included Title X, known as the Family Planning Services and Population Research Act of 1970. Nixon in 1969 said that "no American woman should be denied access to family planning assistance because of her economic condition." Although family-planning funds are found in numerous government funding streams (especially, for example, Medicaid, as well as through Title V mentioned above), Title X formally represents the *only* federal source dedicated solely to reproductive health and family planning. Providers using Title X funds are required to provide contraceptive services to low-income men and women, and clinics such as Planned Parenthood and state/local health departments receive the majority of these funds.[38]

Estimates suggest that in the period from 1980 to the turn of the twentieth century, Title X–supported care prevented approximately 20 million pregnancies.[39] Of course, Title X clinics do not only provide contraceptive services; they also provide low-income women with cancer screening and STD testing, among other things. Since its enacting in 1976, the Hyde Amendment has expressly prohibited federal funds from supporting abortion at these clinics. Still, through other funding sources—including individual women themselves—many of these clinics do provide abortion services.

The bifurcation of reproductive health services and maternal health services—along with insurance coverage decisions based on pregnancy status—has also led to a stark division regarding the physical locations in which women seek reproductive care. In effect, abortion and contraceptive services have largely been cordoned off from maternal and child health care, relegated to the stigmatized silo of reproductive health. This arrangement maintains the realm of maternal health as comparatively "safe" and non-controversial.[40] In an interview, one physician explained that a legacy of the reproductive silos was to push maternal and child health practitioners and policymakers to focus on pregnancy, saying, "I think MCH [maternal and child health] and women's health are the same. I just think that in MCH traditionally we've thought of putting most of our resources on the pregnancy side than [on] health promotion and disease prevention that relates to non-pregnancy. And that's where I think we lost balance. And it's not our fault, because in the United States that's basically been the name of the game when it comes to women" [pediatrician].

The "name of the game when it comes to women" has historically been to divide women's reproductive life course into discrete reproductive moments rather than treating women's health as a full gamut of needs and realities. For example, abortion and pregnancy care are siphoned into distinct worlds—reproductive health and maternal health, respectively—when, in fact, many women need both types of services throughout their reproductive life course. The composition of reproductive care silos, along with the rise of the notion of fetal rights, also arguably stoked the discourse of maternal-fetal conflict in reproductive care,[41] making experts potentially hyperaware of how their work intersects with realms that focus on preventing (or spacing) fetuses and babies and with realms that focus on caring for fetuses and babies.

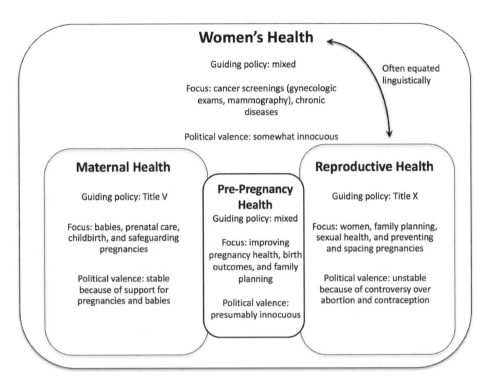

Figure 4. Women's health arena and reproductive silos

Figure 4 above represents the reproductive silos of maternal health and reproductive health. It depicts the ideological and political splits that were so often articulated by the experts I interviewed. These silos guide public-health policy and help determine what types of care are covered and when they are covered. There are multiple kinds of programs that fall within each silo. For example, prenatal care services are clearly within the realm of maternal health, but so is Healthy Start—a program aimed at helping pregnant women, infants, and children. That is, these silos are not entirely representative of medical care or health insurance coverage, but they intersect with both points. Each silo is differentiated by its guiding policy, its focus of programs and care, and its political valence. The idea of the pre-pregnancy care model was to infuse all these programs, to bridge them, and to allow for more overlap.

As is evident from Figure 4, reproductive health and maternal health are generally considered separate silos *within* the broader arena of women's health. But because women's health is often synonymous with reproductive health, and thus incorporates care services like abortion and family planning, experts were loath to use either term. The experts fixated on how a model that includes these worlds could be defined solely in terms of the maternal-health world, or the one that was seemingly not controversial at the time.

The maternal health silo has its federal roots in the early 1900s, but the reproductive health silo finds its federal support at just a little more than four decades old. The latter has consistently been mired in political controversy because of its association with preventing and terminating pregnancies. And although there is certainly some bureaucratic and clinical overlap regarding these worlds of women's health and health care, the ideological divide between the silos is palpable. One ostensibly exists for helping pregnancies and children, the other for preventing pregnancies and children. This divide is entrenched. As one expert explained in an interview: "[Title X] is a group that really wanted [to focus on] family planning and worried about access to contraception. They weren't so interested in the babies; they were interested in the prevention of unwanted babies. And the MCH [maternal and child health] community early on sort of stayed away from them. By and large the MCH community stayed away from family planning" [scientist].

In sum, at an ideological as well as at a bureaucratic and policy level, the silos of reproductive health and maternal health historically have not overlapped. Expressly because of reproductive politics and reproductive silos, experts typically slipped among definitions of women's/reproductive/maternal health, often choosing "pre-pregnancy health" to stand in for all terms, thus potentially avoiding—through semantic finesse—politically contentious topics. Such fluctuating sentiments were illustrative not only of historical schisms but of how experts danced among reproductive definitions and terms, operating as they were within a political and rhetorical cage that has been set up by the "silo-ing" of women's health care in the United States—an apparatus in which only one silo is equated with abortion care.[42] The politics of reproduction and the politics of reproductive semantics shaped language. When experts used the term "women's health," they sometimes referred to everything related to women's health and other times used the term as code for reproductive health or maternal health. The constant slippage of the use of these three different terms in relation to pre-pregnancy care in some ways speaks to how the proponents of this model sought—and seek—to crisscross the boundaries, situating the pre-pregnancy care model as a life-course approach and defying the silos of reproductive health in the United States that treat women's reproductive moments as in need of distinctively different kinds of care that have varying political valences. The next section analyzes how the legacy of reproductive silos infused the work and words of experts charged with defining a new care framework that did not clearly fit the established demarcations.

BRIDGING WORK: REPRODUCTIVE SILOS IN TRANSITION

Boundary issues are ever-present in professional arenas, between medicine and public health,[43] among the reproductive sciences,[44] and within specific reproductive topics. Pre-pregnancy experts, drawn from both medicine and public health, navigated the boundaries presented by the history of reproductive silos in part by advancing a bridging concept— pre-pregnancy care—that would function as a new conceptual container for a host of women's reproductive issues.[45] As Hani Atrash argued, "preconception care is the issue that combines women's health and maternal and child health. It's a women's health issue; it's a pregnancy health issue; it's an infant health issue" [interview]. For many of the experts in these meetings, the need to bridge the worlds of reproductive health and maternal health seemed obvious, but it was not an effortless undertaking. As one expert noted, silos become pronounced during meetings that bring together a professionally diverse set of experts: "You've got two groups of people who come to this meeting. You have people who are interested in women's health. You have people who are interested in the health of babies. And they duke it out. They fight unbelievably at these meetings. I mean, this is not a friendly set of meetings" [scientist].

Some experts entered the CDC meetings not only with the reproductive silos in mind but also with confusion as to which silo they would be addressing. For instance, as one expert was called into the CDC meetings, she wondered what the activity might mean for the women's health world. Given the reproductive silos, she said that she made a conceptual effort expressly to understand how exactly a women's health framework that was not clearly within established reproductive boundaries would fit within the realm of maternity care: "I thought . . . Did I see [pre-pregnancy care] as appropriate within maternal and child health? And I did. It certainly made sense that if you only cared for a woman's health during the period of nine months when she was pregnant, that you were not going to make very much progress. Whereas, if you would pay attention to those critical points along the life course and make interventions there, you would potentially impact positively that health outcome. So, it just made sense" [clinician].

Participants in the CDC meetings—even those who initially were not necessarily on board with couching women's health in terms of maternity—conceded that it was the way to make progress, as this expert did. The tensions between the groups characterized as "for babies" and the groups characterized as "for women" were reportedly still felt, but the respondents for the most part believed in the ability to bring the groups together through the pre-pregnancy concept. The same scientist who explained that groups "duke it out" at these meetings told me in an interview: "I think [pre-pregnancy care] is well-liked because it unites a lot of different factions. It does bring some unity to some of the fights that had existed in the past—family planning versus maternal-child health."

According to the experts I spoke with, pre-pregnancy care indeed traverses divisive historical, political, and ideological boundaries—intentionally so. Specifically, the separation in women's health care was described as one that inevitably would be bridged by a concerted shift toward a clinical and health-promotion framework—the pre-pregnancy care model—that treats non-pregnant women of reproductive age as eligible for expanded health services. For instance, Hani Atrash, the CDC lead on pre-pregnancy care, explained that pre-pregnancy care was clearly something that could bridge some of these silos: "Coupling women's health with pregnancy outcomes made [pre-pregnancy care] a little more attractive because you're talking about babies' health and pregnancy health and women's health, and I think one of the biggest advantages of the pre-conception care initiative to me was bringing the two camps—I would say women's health and MCH [maternal and child health]—together" [interview].

In this quote, Dr. Atrash called the reproductive health arena the women's health arena, as did many experts in the interviews. These untidy definitions betrayed the ongoing split system of the reproductive silos. Dr. Atrash has worked across boundaries in the past, from reproductive health to birth defects. Even someone like Atrash who regularly traverses these boundaries exhibits how the language was at times stifling. Dr. Atrash also made the point that the CDC's initiative for pre-pregnancy care had the unique ability to bring together the reproductive silos and to bridge the divides with a novel approach: pre-pregnancy care. To undertake this bridging work, experts invoked a policy strategy that echoed maternalist political and social strategies in America to advance women's conditions. In their accounts, this approach was necessary given the political context with which they were faced. Put another way, given the legacy of the reproductive silos and the current state of women's health politics, the cultural toolkit[46] the experts drew on revolved around a strategy of maternalism.

STRATEGICALLY MATERNAL

The cultural and scientific "work" that purportedly had to be done to shift reproductive boundaries was accomplished through the course of promoting women's health in terms of a maternal-health lens. Experts did not use the term "maternalism" in describing their work pertaining to pre-pregnancy care, but their accounts entailed exactly that. By reminding politicians and the public that women's bodies are potentially maternal bodies, maternalism was strategically used by experts to bring enhanced attention to women's needs.

One interviewee explained the policy reality driving this strategic approach: "[Legislators] have very little support for uninsured women until they get pregnant because then it's about the baby. It's not about the mother. . . . But, you know, there's just no general primary care money for women . . . because [women] don't have value unless they've got a belly" [public-health researcher]. In expressly seeking to redefine what maternity care means, those involved in the pre-pregnancy care initiative defined all reproductive-aged women as inhabiting a state of expectant motherhood, thus conflating women's reproductive health care with maternal health care and, by extension then, womanhood with motherhood (essentially creating "a belly").

Following is one prominent expert's explanation of the policy and medical problem with Medicaid and health care coverage for low-income women that prompted the need for a pre-pregnancy model: "If you walked into my clinic, told me you're pregnant. . . . Your services are covered. You can have coverage instantaneously. Why? Because you're pregnant. You know, you're special" [obstetrician]. This expert expanded on the systemic problem of lack of care for non-pregnant women by giving the following hypothetical situation:

> You come into my emergency room, you're twenty-four, you have such heavy periods that you're anemic and you need a blood transfusion and I have to give you four units of blood, and I'm going to send you out the door and you: A) can't pay for the hospital bill that you incurred with those transfusions, and B) you can't pay for the medications that I want to give you so that you don't keep having those heavy menstrual periods, and C) you don't have any insurance of any sort, so you're not going to follow up with anybody later on. And guess what? I'm going to see you again in about ten months with the same problem. But the state doesn't value that woman. Why? She's not pregnant. [obstetrician]

This quote nicely illustrates the problems that many clinicians had with health care coverage in the United States—and what made the pre-pregnancy care model's strategy of combining maternal and reproductive health attractive. Across the board, women historically have received more health care attention and more coverage when they are pregnant than when they are not, indicating the social value placed on women as expectant mothers. As mentioned, prior to the Affordable Care Act, low-income women were only valued by the state (by virtue of receiving comprehensive health care coverage) *when they were pregnant*—meaning, of course, that the state would only allow women to seek consistent health care if they were expecting a baby. Low-income women seeking reproductive care thus long have had spotty health care experiences—some services are covered and others, such as abortion, sometimes are not covered by public health services. As emphasized by most experts I interviewed, women in the United States usually have not received political or health attention *unless* they are framed in terms of their maternal social role. The end-story for most of the experts was one of pragmatism—defining women in whatever way works politically and strategically. Maternalism was one realistic strategy. The pre-pregnancy care framework was erected in part as a political attempt at broad coverage for women's health.

Thus, professionals involved in advocating pre-pregnancy care decidedly played on the social and cultural valuation of *women as mothers* rather than of *women as women*. One distinguished expert revealed the political tension of thinking of women both outside and within the proverbial "box" of maternity in the following way:

> We have been so reluctant in the United States to really elevate the importance of the health of women. And every time we even speak [about doing] it, it's always in the context of pregnancy. No one [seems] to really care about a woman's health unless she is pregnant. I mean if you examine, historically, the policies, once you become pregnant you get a lot of help but prior to that you're sort of out there on your own. And that's a very poor way of looking at it, because I believe that a girl is a mother from the time of her own conception. [pediatrician]

This quote eloquently expresses the problem of defining women in terms of maternity, but the expert responded by suggesting that "a girl is a mother from the time of her own conception." By concurrently criticizing and further evoking the political strategy of maternalism, the sentiment expressed here calls upon women of childbearing age to envision themselves as potentially pregnant.

The refrain of maternity served as a potent argument for the material and rhetorical manifestation of pre-pregnancy care. For instance, one respondent explained: "the problem with just saying 'women's health' is then you're losing the focus on the social interests in pregnancy, whereas pre-conception health helps say that society does have an interest in having healthy children because that's the future of the country" [scientist]. The cultural trope that "healthy women make a healthy country" emerged in this statement; investing in children meant that women's health must be front and center.

Indeed, moral and social connotations of the importance of motherhood factored into the experts' discussion of the pre-pregnancy care framework.

Several respondents indicated that they wanted pre-pregnancy health to become as commonplace and "American" as motherhood itself. For example, in one interview an expert pondered: "How do we figure out how it's going to be taught in schools of public health, and schools of public policy, and other [programs], so that this becomes as 'apple pie' and 'motherhood' as prenatal care has been over the last thirty years, given that it's necessary, but not sufficient" [public-health researcher].

Similarly, when asked by CDC representatives whether she would get involved and back pre-pregnancy care, one participant recalled: "And I said, 'Sure.' You know, how can you turn down apple pie and mom?" [obstetrician]. This glorification of the pre-pregnancy care framework as an extension of maternity and "apple pie" draws on and reifies the cultural priority of motherhood as wholesome goodness and worthy of special attention, which also bolsters a strategy of maternalism.

As mentioned above, in the early twentieth century women used maternalist political discourses and strategies to exert political power; in so doing, "they transformed motherhood from women's primary *private responsibility* into *public policy*."[47] This type of strategy—of linking all things female to potential motherhood—continues today, although now it is led by health experts rather than by civic women. The reason the seemingly anachronistic strategy of pre-pregnancy care appeared as silly, or subversive, to many outside observers was perhaps because it came a century after these early maternalist struggles, and after major advances in women's rights. Women could not vote when Julia Lathrop took over the Children's Bureau as the first female head of a federal agency. By the time of the pre-pregnancy push in the beginning of the twenty-first century, third wave feminism was in full swing and women had long had legal access to abortion and to contraception.

MODULATING MISGIVINGS

It is important to note that experts involved in the CDC's pre-pregnancy care meetings varied considerably with regard to whether they personally adhered to a maternalism ideology. Maternalism emerged as a pragmatic political strategy for all involved in the initiative, but for some it was also a personal and professional philosophy. Others were not so quick to exalt women's maternal status, and expressed concern that the pre-pregnancy care approach could open the gates for a potential reversion back to anachronistic thinking of women as baby-making machines. That is, while expressing allegiance to the framework and promise of pre-pregnancy care, some experts exhibited hesitation about its message.[48] One expert, for instance, explained such concerns: "I do agree that you have to look at the health of the mother before she gets pregnant. I just felt the term was kind of degrading to women almost because it just kind of assumed that ... your life should be spent thinking about getting pregnant" [epidemiologist].

Another respondent expressed similar ambivalences about the conflation of womanhood with maternity, saying in an interview, "You know, to me, that rubric—pre-conception care—just presumes that you are a reproductive being and ... while I think that's important because, you know, clearly women are the childbearers, I always had a little reserve—if you will, concern—in the back of my mind that, you know, 'Geez, we're sending this expectation of pregnancy out to women'" [public-health researcher].

Many of the experts were attuned to the ways in which defining a nebulous "women's health" moment (not being pregnant) in terms of pregnancy ("potentially pregnant") might present undue attention and burden on women. In other words, if women are only defined as important given their potential maternity status, then attention to women *qua* women could fade.

Despite these concerns, and as already detailed in this chapter, experts persisted in making a practical calculation of the women's health arena, repeating a seasoned political strategy associated with promoting women's status in America. The reasoning for this approach hinged on attentiveness to what one interviewee succinctly described as the "real systematic under-investment in women's health" [public-health researcher]. Experts deemed it additionally pragmatic to think of women as potential mothers because most women do get pregnant at some point in their lifetime.[49] In phrasing reminiscent of earlier quotes, another expert said, "it's easier to sell pre-conception or inter-conception care as a way of improving the health of newborns than it is to sell that we ought to take better care of women" [public-health researcher]. A political imperative again comes through in this exchange. As mentioned previously, it was deemed easier to "sell" women's health care if defined in terms of babies. Another respondent explained that the idea of general "women's health" is simply "not going to fly anymore . . . it's become a politicized word and people attribute different baggage and that was always the problem with it in the first place" [obstetrician].

Similarly, Hani Atrash explained:

> We [in pre-pregnancy health meetings] talk about women's health clearly. It is women's health. It is having women being healthy before they get pregnant. Now my answer was we've had women's health programs since 1978, I think, when we started that movement. Every health department, every agency, every office in the United States has an office on women's health. And I say, "We have an office in women's health period." There's no money, there are no programs, there are no resources, there are no activities. We just have the name on the door, just like minority health. Everybody has a minority health office. [interview]

So, although pre-pregnancy health *is* women's health, Atrash argued, there is a political imperative not to call it as such. As this chapter has revealed, experts were politically savvy and also entrepreneurial in their hesitance to call what they deemed a women's health-related agenda "women's health." Because of the acrimonious history of reproductive politics and care in America, experts interested in improving women's health *and* birth outcomes had learned to couch their language only in terms of babies and pregnancies, not necessarily mentioning women or family planning, with the hopes of thereby circumventing any contentious political debate about women's health. Politicians and legislators—according to one expert—"easily turn up their nose at women," but the experts knew that if health and support were "linked to the baby" then they would "have a better chance" at "garnering support" than if they used the "R-word"— meaning "reproductive health"—because "that immediately means abortion" [clinician]. There is a political silencing that takes place around reproductive health in the United States, and it became clear that the political context of our time—especially abortion politics—provided the backdrop for the need to bridge reproductive-care worlds.[50] A solution to pressing population health problems was devised, and everyone—even those who were initially skeptical of the idea—eventually got on board with the tacit coalition.[51] Yet this collaborative big umbrella—the "tacit coalition"[52]—remains, as one expert told me, an "uneasy alliance." He explained: "There was a tension between Title X and Title V and it really hasn't resolved to this very day. I mean, you can hear that the two worlds are just suspicious of each other. Pre-conception, however, is a topic that both of them could get behind" [scientist].

REPRODUCTIVE JUSTICE AND STUBBORN DUALITIES

Maternal and child health, as an organizing concept within the federal government, has its roots in the early twentieth century. Maternal and child health was formed politically as largely separate from family planning and reproductive health. It is this disjuncture between maternal health and reproductive health in the arena of women's health care that has allowed for passionate and ongoing debates over interpretations of pre-pregnancy care and its broader meaning for women and society. The realm of maternal health historically has focused most of its attention on births and babies, and the realm of reproductive health has directed its efforts on women's ability to prevent, delay, or space births and babies. This chapter briefly explores this discordant history of reproductive care and politics in America—that which has entrenched a division between reproductive silos, all the while leaving women on the whole without much support or attention when it comes to comprehensive health care. I argue that it is this history that leavened the pre-pregnancy care framework, moving it from an unfamiliar and speculative idea in the medical literature to a prominent place in public health and policy discussions in the twenty-first century.

Very often, discussions about reproductive rights center on the right *not* to get pregnant or carry a pregnancy to term. But from a reproductive justice framework it is just as important to foster opportunities for individuals to engage in reproduction if and when they want to do so. The right to reproductive health has often been overlooked in general in politics, but even more so when it comes to historically-marginalized population groups, such as African-American women, Native American women, and low-income women.[53] The term "reproductive justice" is relatively new, appearing in the 1990s among feminists of color in advocating for reproductive rights to encompass aspects of "choice" beyond simply abortion and contraception, such as the choice and right to have children and to parent.[54] If, for example, a woman without health insurance lives for years with an untreated disease or infection, and this lack of care impedes her ability to have children in the future, then reproductive justice has not been served. In attempting to expand health care access to all women of reproductive age, pre-pregnancy health experts were perceptively attending to the plight of women who could face hurdles when trying to reproduce, due to a lifetime of discrimination—in short, they were attending to issues of social justice.[55] And yet scholars have warned that focusing on expanded access to health care might not address systemic issues (such as racism) within health institutions—potentially, then, exacerbating the risk of adverse birth outcomes.[56]

The analysis in this chapter complicates the standard narrative that the pre-pregnancy care model is reductionist, but it also brings to the fore ongoing and challenging dualities in the realm of reproductive rights that, to some degree, animate the rest of this book. There have long been divisions within the reproductive-rights community between those whose main goal has been about contraception and medical intervention versus those whose emphasis is on reproductive empowerment. As sociologists Carole Joffe and Jennifer Reich write, it is a "fine, and sometimes confusing, line between viewing [reproductive] services as emancipating or coercive for women."[57] Scholars note that reproductive rights today must be thought of in terms of a triad: the right to mother, the right to contracept, and the right to end a pregnancy[58]—aspects of reproduction that are sometimes pitted against one another in cultural discourse and public policy making.

The idea of pre-pregnancy care was meant to promote the health of *all women* of reproductive age. Tensions no doubt were brought about by the attempt to use pre-pregnancy health as code for "women's health"— as experts evinced concern that many in the women's health care arena worried about couching women in terms of potential motherhood. But, as most of the experts believed, using semantic stand-ins for "women's health" was crucial to pursue comprehensive women's health. That is, the work they were doing captured a basic commitment to women's health, even if it largely ignored abortion. At the same time, the experts relied on an age-old strategy of maternalism, enveloping and employing strict ideas about the relationship between potential motherhood and reproductive risk. Maternalism, or defining women's needs in terms of maternity, was seemingly the only pathway that made sense, politically and culturally.

In the end, the pre-pregnancy care approach challenged the long-held categorical burden of pregnancy as the entry point into comprehensive health care for U.S. women. In turn, this maternalism strategy set up a discourse of what I call *anticipatory motherhood* whereby the new categorical imperative for maternity care is no longer "pregnant" but "potentially pregnant." The ethic of anticipatory motherhood exhorts women to minimize health risks in anticipation of inevitable pregnancies.[59] Pre-pregnancy is a framework, then, that envisions all women of childbearing age as maternal bodies.

As made clear in Chapter 3 and in the present chapter, the status of "expectant" and "potential" motherhood has long been part of policy and medical strategies related to women's health care provision. In an analysis of women's health care in the United States, Carol Weisman writes, "a distinctive feature of many of the enacted gender-specific public policies related to women's health is a focus on maternity, that is, on the health of women as mothers or potential mothers."[60] In efforts to improve maternal and child health over the past century, women often have been deemed as the party responsible for fostering improvements in birth outcomes. Women as mothers usually are depicted as keepers of the nation's health, and as being responsible for social order in addition to children's health outcomes.[61] Maternalist health strategies, in how they couch women in terms of their maternity function, could have either positive or adverse consequences on women's social status, as maternalist politics highlight important contradictions in debates over women's agency in society.[62] Such policy making thus has the advantage of "offer[ing] special benefits to women, but it may also perpetuate gender-based disadvantages."[63] A reproductive justice frame not only attends to gender-based inequalities but also accounts for class and race disadvantages, among others. And so a pressing question for reproduction scholars is how to think through a potentially uneasy alliance between notions of reproductive justice and maternalism. That is to say, how to pursue feminist advances amid ongoing reproductive injustice in our society is an enduring concern.[64]

By couching the new care model in terms of pregnancy, rather than general "health," experts were pursuing the political work of avoiding contentious debates over abortion and family planning within the women's health arena. Pregnancy health and the health of babies, experts argued, are politically more acceptable than advocating for women's health—or men's health, for that matter. In so doing, they were drawing on a long history of maternalism in U.S. health care and policy making. It is this categorization, many have argued, that achieves results. Maternalism historically has worked for expanding women's services and continues to be entrenched, shaping how experts and policy makers understand and define women's needs and the needs of babies. Pre-pregnancy care emerged doing as much political and cultural work as it was doing medical and public health work. Although this chapter and the previous one revealed that there was variation in the intent and meaning of the emergent pre-pregnancy care model among experts—as at times it appeared to be progressively justice-oriented and at times appeared to be stubbornly regressive—any difference became leveled in health-promotion materials. Such is the focus of the next two chapters.

5 Get a Reproductive Life Plan!

PRODUCING THE ZERO TRIMESTER

Anyone who has had any experience with childbirth—whether as an expectant mother or as a partner, friend, or family member—likely knows about the book *What to Expect When You're Expecting*. It is a classic, to be sure, regardless of whether one reads or heeds any of the guidance inside it. The popular advice manual even sparked a 2012 Hollywood movie with the same title, starring Jennifer Lopez and Cameron Diaz. Not as many people may know of a more recent iteration of the book, *What to Expect Before You're Expecting*.[1] This version was published after the launch of the CDC's pre-pregnancy care meetings and opened with the following statements: "pregnancy, as you probably know, is nine months long. . . . But is nine months really long enough? . . . It's time to add more months to pregnancy. . . . At least three more months, in fact, for a full year (or even more) of baby making."[2] Explicitly citing the CDC's work in the introduction, the guide's author Heidi Murkoff explained why it is essential for women and their partners to start thinking in an extended trimester framework. Today, as part of this broadened reproductive-risk model, clinicians urge women to draft a "reproductive life plan"—aiming to optimize women's health, aiming to anticipate any risks to future reproduction.

Operationalizing the zero trimester is not just limited to advice books or reproductive life plans. The Kirkman supplement company offers "preconception care vitamins" for both women and men to use to promote optimal health prior to conception. The e.p.t company, probably most famous for its original home pregnancy test, now offers a pre-conception health test that can be purchased over the counter at certain drugstores. The kit tests for vaginal infection, which has been linked to preterm labor (a risk that occurs, of note, *during* pregnancy). Text from the product site reads: "Eliminating vaginal infections prior to conception is as important as taking folic acid or giving up habits like drinking. The e.p.t™ Preconception Health Test helps you easily assess your vaginal health prior to conceiving, is as accurate as a doctor's test, and is clinically proven to be effective . . . visit your doctor for treatment prior to trying to get pregnant." One news release about the product cited the vice president of marketing for the company as saying that "e.p.t was the first to bring the pregnancy test into the home back in 1977, and now we're once again giving women the power to take control of their personal health with the e.p.t Preconception Health Test."[3] This product is marketed as an empowering one for women—one that enables them to take control of their pre-reproductive bodies and to be firmly aware of any problems that might impact a future pregnancy. Although scholars have written eloquently about ethical dilemmas in the rise of pre-conception medical tests[4]—interventions that are usually part of infertility treatments or genetic screenings—health products are increasingly being designed to target *general* optimization of the pre-pregnancy health of all women of reproductive age.

These examples reveal the cultural applicability and marketability of the zero trimester, a time in which reproductive lives can purportedly be assessed, calculated, and rendered less risky. Seemingly, the rise of the pre-pregnancy care framework did more than simply produce a new "common sense" about reproductive risk and bridge reproductive silos; it also helped generate new clinical protocols, new ideas about reproductive responsibility, and new consumer products. That is, as reproductive knowledge and policy were produced, as were medicine, morals, and markets.

This chapter focuses on analyzing the clinical and cultural uptake of the pre-pregnancy care model. It continues to draw on expert interviews, but also examines medical pamphlets, professional literature, public-health campaign materials, media depictions of pre-pregnancy care, and popular books. In so doing, this chapter scrutinizes some of the clinical tools of pre-pregnancy care as well as contemporary cultural discourses surrounding the optimization of pre-pregnancy health and the anticipation of reproductive risk. The following sections highlight the individualized and gendered aspects of pre-pregnancy health ideas and materials to show how pre-pregnancy care reflects a neoliberal health ethos in which women are held individually responsible for optimizing reproduction.

TARGETING "EVERY WOMAN, EVERY TIME"

Pre-pregnancy care advocates have developed what they call an "every woman, every time" approach, in which every clinical encounter a woman has with any physician should be viewed as an opportunity for intervention to render her healthier for a future pregnancy. In a 2003 article that many pre-pregnancy care experts cited as the beginning of the "every woman" method, public-health expert Arlene Cullum argued that "primary care providers who fail to provide preconceptional care to *every woman* of reproductive age during each primary care visit are losing key preventive opportunities."[5] The article went on to state: "It is often assumed that *preconceptional* refers only to women who are planning their first baby, but the term can actually be applied to *any period of time when a potentially fertile woman is not pregnant.*"[6] In discussing this approach, Cullum additionally argued that "every routine primary or specialty care visit and family-planning visit (especially those that include a negative pregnancy test) is an opportunity to provide preconception care for health promotion, disease prevention, and reduction of prenatal and neonatal complications."[7] Dr. Brian Jack also made this argument in the 1990s—that a negative pregnancy test presents an opportune clinical moment for pre-pregnancy intervention.[8]

Thus today it is assumed, according to pre-pregnancy care experts, that "all clinicians who care for women should be aware of the importance of pre-conception health promotion and risk assessment linked to intervention" and that clinicians should ask women of reproductive age about their reproductive plans at every health care visit.[9] One physician I interviewed explained that the "every woman, every time" discussion should come up with any woman who is of childbearing age and is at risk of becoming pregnant. Most experts I spoke with felt that women should think about how their current behaviors—no matter whether they are thinking about getting pregnant—will impact a future pregnancy. With risky women and fragile embryos in mind, the "every woman" approach essentially primes clinicians to take action in the zero trimester—that is, at any time when a woman of reproductive age is not pregnant.[10]

In today's culture, women are urged specifically to see doctors well in advance of pregnancy,[11] and doctors are broadly urged to follow the "every woman, every time" approach. Elaborating the "every woman, every time" approach, Dr. Hani Atrash provided the example of a woman who brings her child in for vaccinations; the pediatrician in this case should ask her whether she is thinking about getting pregnant again: "If she says no, [then ask] 'are you doing anything to avoid getting pregnant?'... If she says yes, [then ask] 'how is your health? Are you taking any medications?' [I]t's like a two-minute discussion and not a special visit" [interview]. In interviews, experts explained that the pre-pregnancy model could be successful if clinicians make "sure that every woman gets everything she needs to have the best pregnancy outcome" [epidemiologist]. The following is one expert's explanation of the importance of this type of approach:

> What I preach to [all medical providers] is given that there's such a high rate of unintended pregnancy in the United States, you can't predict whether that woman of reproductive age that you're seeing today may be pregnant [the next time you see her]. And have you done right by her in your decision-making and your prescriptions, and that kind of stuff? In the event that she's pregnant next time you see her, have you done what you could to encourage her to have a good pregnancy outcome? [An] optimal pregnancy outcome? So, the woman you're seeing in the Emergency Room for a miscarriage, who is someone who is sexually active and fertile, you know, you should be thinking, before you send her home, you should be thinking about, "did she intend to become pregnant?" And if she didn't, have you referred her to the appropriate resources to get the family planning that she needs? [obstetrician]

Essentially, the "every time" approach appeals to clinicians to be more aware of the reproductive status of the women they see in the course of their everyday work and to assist women with family planning. The pre-pregnancy care model certainly exhorts women of reproductive age to be more aware of their reproductive status and intentions, but the success of the model also requires physician initiative. That is, the pre-maternal intensity leveled at women of reproductive age is also aimed at clinicians who treat women of reproductive age.

Some experts I interviewed had mixed feelings about the "every woman, every time" approach to pre-pregnancy care. One respondent said, "I don't think we have yet translated [the model] to respecting every woman who comes into our office, in terms of her desires regarding contraception, her risks, should her contraception not work" [public-policy expert]. And yet some believed that "every woman" was more respectful than "pre-conception;" one expert disliked the term "pre-conception," preferring instead the "every woman" moniker, saying, "I don't think people know what [pre-conception] means. I think the other thing is it tends to subject women to the idea that they're just a vessel to carry babies. And I don't think that women themselves respond to that kind of language as much as they respond to something like 'look good, feel good' or 'every woman'—those kinds of concepts" [nurse]. In another response to the concept of "every woman, every time," one expert explained, "I have no problem with it but I imagine some people might. [Women] might well say, 'this is not what I came to you for'" [public-health researcher].

The approach of "every woman, every time" inculcates reproductive thinking among all women and clinicians in doctors' offices around the country, initiating a conversation about reproductive planning no matter whether the woman came in for a reproduction-related reason. A broken arm might spark a conversation about reproductive planning, for exam-ple. In effect, then, this kind of pre-pregnancy care approach can be per-ceived as one that treats all women as perpetually pre-pregnant.

Nevertheless, the "every woman" approach has had much appeal, sparking major programs in states such as California ("Every Woman California"),[12] Florida ("Every Woman Florida"),[13] and North Carolina ("Every Woman North Carolina")[14]. This concept has also inspired related programs, such as the One Key Question® Initiative launched by the Oregon Foundation for Reproductive Health.[15] This initiative aims to offer pre-conception and contraceptive services as part of an overall goal of reducing unintended pregnancies. The "key" question that a provider is meant to ask a woman of reproductive age is whether she would like to become pregnant in the next year. Similarly, one prominent pre-pregnancy clearinghouse site—Before, Between and Beyond Pregnancy, run by UNC-Chapel Hill and the Preconception Health and Health Care Initiative—offers a toolkit that includes assisting providers in practicing pre-pregnancy care,[16] and one component is also the "vital sign" question of: "Would you like to become pregnant in the next year?" The aim of the toolkit is "to help clinicians reach *every woman* who might someday become pregnant *every time* she presents for routine primary care with efficient, evidence-based strategies and resources to help her achieve: healthier short- and long-term personal health outcomes, increased likelihood that any pregnancies in her future are by choice rather than chance, decreased likelihood of complications if she does become pregnant in the future."[17] Further instantiating "choice" rhetoric might seem empowering but also further individualizes reproductive burden in addition to presenting "choice" as a workable option for all women. In these two "key question" initiatives, the goals are akin and patently obvious: to remind all women of reproductive age that they need to think about their reproductive life plan.[18]

Of course, in practice, asking an individual woman about her reproductive plans might give detailed, useful information about that particular woman's risk status. Conversely, highlighting *every* woman also might involve a strategy that tends to position all women on a similar risk plane, as if risk is equal opportunity, when in fact some women are much more at risk than others. For example, African American women are 2.4 times more likely to experience an infant death by that infant's first birthday than are non-Hispanic white women. Nearly half (46%) of infant deaths to black women are preterm-related complications, as opposed to the 32% of preterm-related infant deaths that occur to non-Hispanic white women.[19] Black women also are more likely to have unintended pregnancies.[20] To the extent that the pre-pregnancy care framework was organized to address adverse birth outcomes and pregnancy planning, it might have been assumed that the framework would pay close attention to such racial disparities, and that, by extension, any clinical operationalization of the framework would have been attuned to reproductive risk by race or other social statuses.

Some professionals have indeed situated the reproductive life plan as an important tool for addressing racial disparities in birth outcomes,[21] and many of the experts I interviewed hoped that pre-pregnancy care would address such disparities directly. The CDC's *MMWR* 2006 publication listed reducing health disparities in pregnancy and birth outcomes as one of its top priorities. Moreover, the CDC's pre-pregnancy health and health care initiative included much activity around addressing inequalities in health-care coverage,[22] and inequalities in access to comprehensive health care is often mentioned in pre-pregnancy care research publications. Some experts I interviewed thought that pre-pregnancy care would have a "tremendous impact" [public-health researcher] on racial health disparities, while others thought the evidence for this was "really thin" [scientist]. And yet, several experts with whom I spoke revealed that the CDC meetings did not focus on health disparities to the level they had expected they would. One obstetrician revealed embarrassment at not taking health disparities more seriously sooner in the process of forging the pre-pregnancy care framework, and another respondent explained that the CDC initiative needed to work on its attention to disparities and inclusivity:

> But I think . . . that we need to be, [to] assure, that we're more inclusive of people from all socioeconomic classes, and that we're representative when we have select panels, and other things. So I think that's something we try to be cognizant of. So there wasn't always complete agreement [on the CDC's initiative]. And there's always an interesting thing in health, in public health . . . do you take a broader approach that reaches everybody, or do you focus in on areas where you see distinct disparities in outcomes? And how do you balance those things? When you look at infant mortality, it often is an African American issue, in most communities. [public-policy expert]

This quote carefully navigates the framing of population health interventions as either universal ones or targeted ones. Several experts went further and worried that their work would actually increase the racial gap in pregnancy-related health measures. Following is an excerpt from an interview that reflects a focus on the underlying, fundamental causes of risk:[23]

> As it stands right now there are some who believe that [pre-pregnancy care] could actually exacerbate health disparities. And the reason is because the women most likely to get pre-conception [care] now are women who have resources—women who have access. . . . But I think [pre-pregnancy care] can address health disparities if we make sure that everyone is afforded an opportunity to receive pre-conception care. . . . And a problem with that is unintended pregnancy, you know: the women who are more likely to plan their pregnancy—they are the ones who are more likely to benefit from pre-conception care right now. And so if that's the case, then there may be some disparities. But if we can insure that across the board every woman gets pre-conception care then I think it does have an opportunity to address disparity. [scientist]

Others were skeptical of the pre-pregnancy model's ability to combat infant mortality, especially disparities in infant mortality, as in this interviewee's statement: "I think [pre-pregnancy care] left out some very fundamental pieces, because . . . if you're looking at pre-conception care or pre-conception health as improving the birth outcomes from a general population [perspective], sure. If you're looking at it as an intervention in terms of mortality rates, which for the most part for this country means African American, the answer [about its effectiveness is] 'no'" [public-health researcher].

Dorothy Roberts has written that, especially when reproductive matters are concerned, American culture tends to value individual choice over social justice.[24] An individual-level intervention like "every woman, every time" appears to highlight individual actions, choices, and desires, which might on the surface appear helpful but, at the same time, does not target root changes or social justice. If every woman is optimized and every risk anticipated, certain population groups still will be at disproportionate risk due to other underlying causes, such as pollution, structural racism, lack of access to quality, stable health care, family planning services, or nutritional foods. What does this individualized approach to a population health problem look like in practice? This chapter now turns to discussion of how individualized and universal risk is further institutionalized in clinical settings.

REPRODUCTIVE LIFE PLANS AND INDIVIDUALIZING REPRODUCTIVE BURDEN

As discussed throughout this book, the pre-pregnancy care approach is not aimed solely at improving birth outcomes. A critical goal of the model is also to reduce unintended pregnancies. One of the main ways in which pre-pregnancy care has been operationalized is through what experts label a "reproductive life plan," or a clinical assessment of reproductive intentions and reproductive health risks.

Several of the experts I interviewed credited Merry-K. Moos with the idea of the reproductive life plan. Moos, a nurse practitioner and faculty member in the OB/GYN department at UNC, published articles (mentioned in previous chapters) that were among some of the earliest ones calling for greater attention to pre-pregnancy care in the medical literature. A pioneering study conducted by Moos and colleagues in the 1990s found that a pre-conceptional health promotion program resulted in a higher rate of intendedness in subsequent pregnancies.[25] Thus, family planning has long been part and parcel of the modern pre-pregnancy care framework, and it animates the examples of reproductive life plans on present display. Any type of anticipated biographical narrative counts as a reproductive life plan, as is evident in examples provided below. An individual might report never wanting children, desiring children after achieving certain goals, or anticipating reproduction right around the corner. Whatever the "plan," the underlying message is that the individual presumably owns, in some way or another, the blueprint for her reproductive future—and should act accordingly.

In 2006, Moos provided one clear example of a "reproductive life plan," one which "would specifically invite women to actively consider their current desires regarding childbearing." It consisted of the following questions:

- Do you plan to have any (more) children?
- How many children do you hope to have?
- How long do you plan to wait until you (next) become pregnant?
- How much space do you plan to have between future pregnancies?
- What do you plan to do to avoid pregnancy until you are ready to become pregnant?
- What can I do today to help you achieve your plan?[26]

Moos and other experts interested in developing the reproductive life plan were no doubt influenced by the belief that "the only opportunity to prevent unintended pregnancy is before conception."[27] As discussed in the previous chapters, the unintended pregnancy rate has remained high over time, especially as compared to the rate in other industrialized countries. The idea of a reproductive life plan was developed with the intention to empower individuals to, again, move from "chance" to "choice," in the words of pre-pregnancy care proponents.[28]

This sentiment was evinced in the interviews I conducted, as well as in the meetings and webinars that I attended. Experts explained that unintended pregnancies are associated with the higher likelihood of abortion, late entry to prenatal care, and an increased risk of low birth weight. And those with whom I spoke believed, for the most part, that the reproductive life plan tool was helpful, as illustrated by the following explanation: "[The] reproductive life plan is useful and interesting because it sort of helps people think through . . . what intendedness means or when they want to get pregnant or, you know, when they really don't care whether they do or not or whatever" [epidemiologist]. In discussing the utility of a reproductive life plan in the context of pre-pregnancy care, another expert similarly focused on planning pregnancies: "I think the big, the first, step to pre-conception care is getting women to try and develop reproductive life plans and really think about when and how they get pregnant. . . . So, I think that's the first step, kind of thinking about making more pregnancies planned pregnancies" [epidemiologist].

In an interview, another respondent also endorsed reproductive planning and timing and, in so doing, emphasized contraceptive counseling: "To me, the first step of pre-conception health is having a planned pregnancy . . . or optimally timing your pregnancy. And so for women who are not intending pregnancy . . . part of pre-conception counseling would be finding out what birth control method is most appropriate for them" [scientist].

The tools for pre-pregnancy care have been designed according to the logic that healthy women have healthy babies, and part of the construction of "healthy" is predicated on the idea of being prepared and organized when it comes to family planning. Addressing every woman every time she has a clinical encounter is ideally facilitated if the woman has a reproductive life plan in her pocket, or if she has answers to questions like the ones outlined by Moos above. Indeed, "every woman" clinical guidelines usually recommend that women (and often men, too) draft a such a plan. The following is an excerpt from the Every Woman North Carolina reproductive life planning site: "So, if you agree that making plans for your future family is important, how do you get started? To begin, you can ask yourself these questions: Do I want to have children someday? If no or not sure, what are my plans for making sure I do not become pregnant? If yes, how many would I like to have? How old do I want to be when I become a mother? How many years do I want to have in between children?"[29]

These questions are intended to direct a woman's conversations with her clinical providers. Similarly, the CDC lists examples of individuals' reproductive life plans on its website, and included are the following scenarios that women, and sometimes men, of reproductive age have used to summarize and illustrate their plans:

- I've decided that I don't want to have any children. I will find a good birth control method. Even though I don't want to have children, I will talk to my doctor about how I can be healthier.

- I'm not ready to have children now because I want to finish school first. I'll make sure I use effective birth control and protect myself from sexually transmitted diseases every time I have sex. Some day, I think I'd like to have two or three children about 2 years apart. Before I get pregnant, I will talk to my doctor about losing weight and eating healthy.

- I want to have children when I've saved some money. My partner has diabetes so, when it's time, I'll encourage her to see her doctor to make sure her body is ready for pregnancy. In the meantime, we're taking really good care of ourselves just for us.

- I might want to have children one day, but I'm not sure right now. For now I'm not going to have sex. Even though I'm not ready to have kids yet, I'm going to talk with my doctor about how I can be as healthy as possible.

- I am in a good relationship and I'm pretty healthy. I want to stop using birth control and try to get pregnant. I'm going to talk to my doctor to find out what I can do to have a healthy pregnancy.

- I've had two kids, and they were only a year apart. Both times, it just happened. I want to have another kid before I turn 36, but I want to wait at least 2 years. I'll talk to my doctor about birth control. This time, I'm going to make sure I get pregnant only when I want to.

- My partner and I are ready to have a child, but we'll need to use a sperm bank or fertility service to get pregnant. I'll make sure I'm in good health and financially stable before we use those services.[30]

When should such plans begin to foment in individuals' minds? According to some experts I interviewed, the reproductive life plan "should really start in the preteen years" [public-health researcher], and many of the pre-pregnancy health recommendations target young people, as some of the materials listed above undoubtedly do. Another expert explained to me that "continuing to work with young adults and teens about . . . life planning is important," while lightheartedly acknowledging that schools and teen environments are not the "most conducive environment to really be thinking about your life plan" [public-health researcher].

As a prominent example of how reproductive planning among teenagers has become an integral component of pre-pregnancy care, the March of Dimes hosts an educational curriculum for teachers and youth volunteers, titled "Pregnancy is Now 12 Months!" The website for the program explains, "Can pregnancy be 12 months long? Yes, if you include planning as a necessary component, sort of a trimester of its own." It goes on to clarify, "The program refers to the idea that to have a healthy mom, a healthy pregnancy, and a healthy baby, forethought is key. Ideally, every pregnancy would include at least three months of planning followed by nine full months of gestation."[31] The March of Dimes essentially discusses the zero trimester as an actual "trimester of its own," emphasizing that a responsible pregnancy would include abundant consideration ahead of time. Young women are primed to think that life without a reproductive plan could mean that the health of their future children is at stake.

A reproductive life plan has been positioned in the pre-pregnancy care model as part of the bigger trend toward anticipatory screening in health care mentioned in Chapter 1 and Chapter 3, and such tools have been highlighted as a potentially effective way to advise women with chronic diseases or unsafe behaviors about their reproductive risks.[32] One interviewee described the reproductive life plan as "a piece of this story that I think we're trying to promote, to be thinking kind of proactively about, you know, if you're single, but anticipate sometime in the future being in a relationship and wanting to conceive, or if you're in a relationship, and even if you're not currently planning to conceive, that you still see this as something that ought to be in your awareness, just like getting a tetanus shot, or a flu shot, or getting a mammogram" [physician]. In this way, the reproductive life plan was depicted as simply another tool in the litany of anticipatory health practices that people are urged to engage in today. Life-plan materials intimate that it is no longer culturally acceptable to "just get pregnant," but rather to make sure that the body is *ready* for pregnancy.[33] Even though many women do not have a distinct reproductive life plan,[34] this approach might work for women; one program found that women responded more enthusiastically to a "reproductive life plan" tool than to general messages about the importance of pre-pregnancy health.[35] The reproductive life plan tool has recently expanded to become a Web-based technique to help reduce unintended pregnancies.[36]

Asking women to reflect on a set of life-plan questions has infiltrated discourse about pregnancy health in the popular press as well. Women's magazines now tend to highlight the anticipation of the reproductive future, as in this quote from *Shape Magazine*: "as more women delay pregnancy until later in life, it's important to get the facts early on so your body is ready for [a] baby when you finally do decide you want one."[37] In *Parents Magazine*, a "preconception checklist" was published in the November 2010 issue, and it included a long list of tasks to undertake before getting pregnant: "Whether you're actively trying or just thinking about getting pregnant, you can take steps now to make the experience as healthy and joyful as possible." It further instructed readers to "Print and carry this handy checklist to keep track of your efforts."[38] The website of *Parents Magazine* also highlighted a slideshow of foods to initiate a "Pre-Conception Diet Makeover."[39]

Notably, much of the literature in women's magazines related to pre-pregnancy discussions narrates fears about infertility and weight-gain—inserting worries in readers' minds about how pre-pregnancy behaviors might harm a future pregnancy. In 2014, *Women's Health* magazine highlighted "4 Foods You Should Avoid Now If You Want to Get Pregnant Later,"[40] and has included other headlines in its pages, such as "Want a Baby Someday? How to Preserve Your Fertility" with the subheading, "If you're thinking about getting pregnant later in life, you need to take certain steps right now to help keep your body in peak baby-making shape."[41] In February 2014, *Redbook* published a piece titled "The Pregnancy Health Crisis No One's Talking About," which covered the risk of not losing pregnancy weight *prior to* the next pregnancy. It stated that weight is "a health risk that can affect women and their children for the rest of their lives."[42] Reproductive planning projects have come into vogue—and largely appear to be privileged projects in which perhaps only some women have the time or resources to engage.[43]

As part of this trend, women and couples are urged to buy volumes devoted to how best to improve pre-pregnancy health. As mentioned at the beginning of this chapter, Heidi Murkoff, of the famed pregnancy book *What to Expect When You're Expecting*, drew on the momentum of the CDC's endorsement of pre-pregnancy care to write a new iteration of the self-help book, *What to Expect Before You're Expecting: The Complete Preconception Plan*. In the text, Murkoff explains how important a pre-pregnancy health care visit is and how to eat well and get in shape before becoming pregnant. The first chapter from this book, "Prepping Before You're Expecting," starts off by saying, "Are you gearing up for a pregnancy? Preparing for baby making isn't only about tossing your birth control (though you'll need to do that), charting your ovulation (you'll probably want to do that), and heading to bed (you'll be happy to do that). It's also about getting your body . . . into tip-top shape."[44] The book includes numerous topics such as eating well prior to conception, understanding ovulation, addressing fertility challenges if they arise, pre-conception genetic screening, and pre-pregnancy immunizations, among other things.

Murkoff's book states that it was influenced by the CDC's initiative, but there were earlier publications that picked up on the growing pre-pregnancy health trend in the medical literature in the late 1980s and early 1990s, including *Before You Conceive: The Complete Prepregnancy Guide*[45] and *The Twelve-Month Pregnancy: What You Need to Know Before You Conceive to Ensure a Healthy Beginning for You and Your Baby*.[46] A book published in 1980 titled *Pre-Parenting: A Guide to Planning Ahead*[47] shows that "prepregnancy" literature existed even prior to the more current wave of pre-pregnancy advice books, although the book's text was less in the vein of contemporary literature that focuses on preparing and optimizing the body.

It was rather focused on how to make decisions about becoming a parent in light of social and cultural changes. Written in response to contraceptive and legal advances that allowed for greater reproductive choice in the 1970s, the authors wrote that "the availability of contraception and abortion requires that we must make decisions about having children that were once dictated mainly by chance."[48] "Health considerations" in this book were largely concerned with birth control.

To contrast this 1980 text with more recent publications is to grasp that the current pre-pregnancy health guides emphasize not just family planning but also the optimization of women's health to provide a healthier basis for future pregnancies. A good example of this sentiment is the book *Before Your Pregnancy: A 90-Day Guide for Couples on How to Prepare for a Healthy Conception*, first published in 2002 and then again in 2011.[49] The introduction was titled "Don't Just Conceive: Preconceive!" The book covered everything from lifestyle habits (caffeine, drugs) to stress, environmental safety, genetics, nutrition, exercise, and infertility. It was aimed at enhancing the health of *all* women of reproductive age who might want a baby someday.

Additionally, Michael Lu's *Get Ready to Get Pregnant: Your Complete Prepregnancy Guide to Making a Smart and Healthy Baby*,[50] published in 2009, focused on preparing for pregnancy with proper nutrition, stress resilience,[51] and environmental health awareness. Lu is a known star in the maternal and child health world; he previously was the director of UCLA's Preconception Care Clinic and has continued to be a national leader in the field. In this book, he devoted a chapter to explaining what pre-pregnancy care is and when a woman should see a doctor for this kind of care (answer: "the sooner, the better").[52] Topic number one on what should be discussed in a pre-pregnancy health care visit is the reproductive life plan, which Lu defined as "a set of personal goals about having (or not having) children based on your personal values and resources, and a plan and timeline to achieve those goals."[53]

Other health materials designed for public consumption also position the ability to have a future healthy baby squarely in women's reproductive foresight. In a March of Dimes Prematurity Campaign poster that featured the Latina pop singer Thalía, she says, "I'm not pregnant . . . but I want my 9 months . . . someday." She goes on to explain, "In the meantime, I'll do

everything I can to make sure that when I become pregnant, my baby will
be born healthy. More and more babies are born too early and those who
survive may have serious health problems. *No one knows why some babies
are born prematurely.* But we do know there are things a woman can do,
even before pregnancy, to help give her baby a full 9 months. The March of
Dimes recommends getting a *preconception checkup* before you get pregnant" (emphasis added).[54]

This message indicates that any risk to any potential fetus should be—
and can be—mitigated. In this poster text, Thalía expresses she "will do
everything [she] can to make sure" that her future baby will be healthy.
What follows on the poster is a list of "preconception checkup" topics for
her to address with her doctor. The message text conceded that "no one
knows why some babies are born prematurely" but then continued to list
all the things a woman and her doctor should try to do to prevent it. This
"responsibility message" is disconcerting given the statistic that many
neonatal deaths occur to otherwise healthy women,[55] and it serves as
another example of the individualized spirit of reproductive planning
discourse.

The strategy invoked in "reproductive life plans" is characteristic of what
Foucault discussed as projects or technologies of the self.[56] The emphasis on
future pregnancy risks is "part of a broader development in contemporary
subjectivity: that which presents one's life and self as a 'planning project.'"[57]
According to these materials, it is up to women to come up with their reproductive life strategy, arrange their lives accordingly, and stick to their plan.
Only then, the discourse intimates, will women have an optimal shot at a
healthy pregnancy one day. It is worth considering that pre-pregnancy care
is hyper-planning to such an extent that it might render active planning
obsolete. That is, the reproductive life plan and other pre-pregnancy tools
are manifestly aimed at improving intentions, but the latent aim is to change
lifestyles. If one's life is lived in a pre-pregnant fashion, one can "safely" get
pregnant anytime, even without an overt plan in place.

We return to this point again in Chapter 6, but for now it is notable that
an individualized "project" approach to reproduction is reminiscent of the
"risk society" of late modernity.[58] Indeed, contemporary risk deals with
future occurrences, "as related to present practices—and the colonizing
of the future therefore opens up new settings of risk, some of which are

institutionally organized."[59] The reproductive life plan is about optimization and anticipation of risk, and it is an established tool for clinical practice.[60] According to the pre-pregnancy care model, women must engage in individualized projects to alter their lifestyles and offset any and all future risks to their future pregnancies.

GENDERING REPRODUCTIVE RESPONSIBILITY

Why did the pre-pregnancy health initiative promote this idea of "every woman, every time" and the practice of asking all women of reproductive age questions about reproductive life plans and about all potential risks? As typified by the following quote from an expert I interviewed, "nurturance" is one major factor:

> Well, in many ways, I think [pre-pregnancy care is] about women nurturing their bodies, so that when they're ready, they can nurture another body! You know, and be part of a creative process that they're uniquely designed to do! That would be a favorable outcome. And so, me, I've always thought . . . it's a natural process; it's a nurturing process, and if we could be kinder and more mindful of the stewardship of our own bodies, so that we're prepared to do that for another life? . . . That that would be a positive thing for both [mother and baby], and a good outcome for both. That's sort of how I think about it. We all have challenges. I mean, we all have different habits that don't set us up well for that! Or hang-ups, or addictions, or things that challenge our own ability to self-nurture, let alone have a body that's able to nurture another life. [scientist]

The sentiment about the need to nurture expressed in this excerpt reveals an individualized burden for the health of one's own body and the future health of another. This burden was often, perhaps unsurprisingly, supplied with gendered cultural assumptions about nurturance, situated as applying only (or mainly) to women's bodies. Pre-pregnancy health promotional materials focus largely on women, and the majority of medical journal articles and popular articles on pre-pregnancy health highlight women's bodies and behaviors. Indeed, most of the clinical and cultural pre-pregnancy health advice has been aimed at women directly, despite findings from population studies that about 60% of men are in need of pre-conception care.[61] Political scientist Cynthia R. Daniels has written that men often are ignored in social and scientific discussions of fetal harm. "While men's physical distance from gestation creates the illusion that men's relation to fetal health is tangential, in reality, a man's use of drugs or alcohol or his exposures to toxins long before conception can profoundly affect the health of the children he fathers."[62] Moreover, sociologists have revealed that scientists and clinicians tend to overlook male factors in discussing pre-pregnancy risk factors in reproduction.[63] Social policy as well often designates women as the sole bearers of fetal safety.[64] And in popular portrayals of pre-conception harm in U.S. newspapers, mothers are defined as "bad," and dads as "blameless."[65] If women's environments and health behaviors prior to conception contribute to the quality of early fetal development, then we must wonder how men's environmental exposures and social behaviors prior to conception—that is, both their biological and behavioral characteristics—impact the well-being of the future fetal environment.

In this vein, some pre-pregnancy health scholars have attended to the risks men pose to future fetuses.[66] And discussions about men did emerge in some of my interviews with experts and in some of the materials I reviewed. For instance, a few experts included men when touting the importance of reproductive plans: "It's not just the woman's reproductive life plan [that matters], but the man has a reproductive life plan as well" [nurse]. When experts sought to broaden the "every woman" approach, men were discussed in terms of their role as part of a couple; as Hani Atrash explained: "I agree with [every woman, every time]. I would go beyond that—I would say every person every time because I don't want just to focus on the woman. I think we're talking about couples and there's always the role of the man in the picture" [interview].

Thus, pre-pregnancy health experts made it known that they had thought about integrating men more directly into pre-pregnancy care, even though much of the attention in pre-pregnancy care is on women. One expert explained in an interview that men should also fully engage in the "reproductive life plan" activities:

> And I would also really, really, really want us to stop putting it all on women. I want us to start talking to men and boys and saying, "When do you want to

get somebody pregnant? What do you want for your future? How are you going to support your partner when she does get pregnant." . . . You know I just feel like everything—especially with pregnancy or even family planning—is always put on the women. I think we really, really, really need to kind of shift that conversation [and] understand that pregnancy happens in a partnership. [epidemiologist]

Although this respondent went beyond a frame that focuses only on women, the expectation that pregnancy happens in a partnership belies the fact that there are socioeconomic differences in the extent to which pregnancies happen in a viable or recognizable "partnership." In interviews, other experts listed the specific ways that men pose risks to future pregnancies; for example: "We need to really try to engage men in the arena of pre-conception care. Men who drink, men who use drugs, men who smoke all pose risks to a healthy pregnancy. And, you know, even if they're not the ones who get pregnant, it's still a two-person act and really engaging the boys and men around sexual health, sexual responsibility, and the full spectrum of care and preparedness—planning for eventual pregnancy—is absolutely essential" [public-health researcher].

At the same time that most respondents explained that men are important to think about, in the end they felt that it remained most essential to focus on risks that women pose to future pregnancies, telling me that "you know, ultimately, ninety-eight percent of the evidence suggests it's intrauterine environment that's the most important thing" [obstetrician]. Likewise, Hani Atrash explained the reasons why the label had to be "every *woman*, every time": "the problem is couples don't come together to the health-care system every time, so that's why [the slogan is] every woman, every time. We unfortunately put the load and the burden on the woman not on the man. But again [it] goes back to [the fact that] women are the people who get pregnant" [interview].

Similarly, the popular self-help books on pre-pregnancy care mentioned above include "couples" and usually devote a chapter to men. For instance, *The 90-Day Guide for Couples on How to Prepare for a Healthy Conception* includes a chapter on men, arguing that men, too, should plan at least ninety days in advance of conception to produce vibrant and healthy sperm through healthy eating and exercise, among other things. Dr. Lu's book on making a smart and healthy baby also devotes a whole chapter to men, providing a 10-step plan to get ready for paternity. The first step is to make a reproductive life plan; steps 2 through 6 are about making good sperm, and 7 through 10 are about supporting the pregnant woman.[67] Yet, men are the focus in only one chapter, and when mentioned elsewhere the assumption tends to be that it is the woman who is reading the book.

Additionally, discussions around men's pre-conception health appear in popular magazines; however, such mentions are less about general health optimization than about making a pregnancy happen in the first place. For example, a *Men's Health* article titled "5 Reasons She's Not Getting Pregnant" highlighted all the behavioral changes a man could take to improve the chances of a healthy conception, such as quitting smoking, eating better foods, and keeping computers off his lap.[68]

Thus, while most experts in this study said that men were important, it was largely a symbolic gesture. Experts and advice books were likely to state that *couples*—usually defined as a man and a woman—are important when it comes to achieving a healthy pre-pregnancy environment, and yet men still have received very little formal attention in this framework. Further, to the extent that women's reproductive health care might be extended through a pre-pregnancy care model, men's access to reproductive care generally has been disregarded.

This gendered focus in pre-pregnancy care means that a pre-maternal discourse is not met with a parallel pre-paternal discourse. Despite mentioning men here and there, most popular materials (as was the case in the medical literature) specifically advise women to remain responsible and vigilant future mothers, without always also advising men to act accountably as future fathers. Critics have warned that the potential "psychological effect of such advice is to have women thinking as mothers well before they conceive."[69] One CDC poster from 2009 reveals a reproductive responsibility message that is highly gendered, urging women to be attentive to their reproductive futures: "You may not be ready to have a baby, but your body's been preparing for years." The fine print explained: "You have lots to do before motherhood. But make sure to take folic acid today—and every day. Whether you get it in a pill by itself, in a multivitamin, or in foods like breakfast cereals, breads and pastas, this essential B vitamin helps prevent some serious birth defects in babies."[70] The strategy in this poster revolved around the expectation of motherhood and the expected individual preparation for such a life event.

Popular magazines convey similar messages regarding a maternal imperative. For example, a *Shape* article about infertility emphasized the importance of keeping a fertile body ready to go: "New research reveals that every woman should take steps today to protect her fertility, regardless of whether she has babies on the brain or can't imagine being a mom for a while (or ever). This step-by-step plan will not only help you have a healthy family, it'll keep you strong and fit for years to come."[71] *Essence* magazine targeted future motherhood clearly in an article titled "How to Prepare for Pregnancy Now (Even Though You're Nowhere Close to Actually Being Pregnant!)": "Regardless of your status, your future children are already living inside of you. As women, we are born with all the eggs we will ever have, with up to 2 million immature follicles tucked away in our infant ovaries. For that reason we should prepare now for future parenthood. First things first: It's not all about age."[72]

Several pre-pregnancy care experts I interviewed worried about such messages that might induce guilt among women, as the following quote reveals:

> [Pre-pregnancy care] smacks of "uterism" as they call it—you know, we're only for our uteruses. And it's also—it can be blaming, you know, for women. Well, you know, [what if] we give this [advice] and [women] don't do anything with it. Are you a bad person? And, your baby's not healthy because you didn't take a vitamin? . . . We ran into a lot of challenges with folic acid in terms of, like I said, trying to shift the message away from pregnancy and also to be careful that you wouldn't somehow make a woman feel—whose baby had spina bifida—that she was a bad mother because she didn't take it, you know what I mean? And maybe she didn't know about it or maybe she was genetically predisposed and she just took four hundred micrograms and she needed the higher dose. And so I think that's why . . . I had run into that with folic acid the hard way like we mostly do, you know what I mean? . . . [W]hen you step in . . . and then you find out you've done something completely unintentionally and someone felt really bad. [public-health researcher]

This respondent was particularly thoughtful about how pre-pregnancy messages could potentially make women feel undue blame. Another public-health expert worried about how to prime pre-pregnancy health messages: "How do you make a marketing campaign that really gets across what we want to say without making women feel like we're expecting them to have babies, you know? How do you take into account every woman's personal situation and background in a marketing campaign?" In highlighting gendered expectations of women and potential maternal guilt, some experts were combating the neoliberal tendency in the pre-pregnancy care framework to individualize reproductive risk. Yet, despite such reflective sentiments from experts, pre-pregnancy health campaigns continued to tout these neoliberal messages, as Chapter 6 further details.

PRODUCING NEOLIBERAL REPRODUCTIVE BODIES

Neoliberalism is a dominant political and economic ideology today that promotes deregulation, entrepreneurship, and privatization.[73] It is an ideology that positions all outcomes as equally possible and equally earned, regardless of situation or context. It therefore is a system that holds individuals fully responsible for their conditions and ailments.[74] This framework has permeated the health realm, in both health programs and messaging, most clearly by emphasizing the role of individual behavior for health outcomes.[75]

The idea of "every woman, every time" highlighted in this chapter is illustrative of the neoliberal ethos in the sense that all women of reproductive age are set up as being "at risk" of experiencing a future adverse reproductive outcome, and the success of the approach hinges on physicians asking women to be aware of and articulate their reproductive plans. Scholars have argued that placing biological or individual-level emphasis on health risks and remedies potentially masks health inequalities that are in part due to social factors.[76] If, for instance, the marketing of pre-pregnancy tools and health behaviors only reach and impact middle-class America, then the model might not come close to achieving its goals of improving reproductive outcomes at the population level.

With the reproductive life plan, a neoliberal individual responsibility culture is also on display, one that is highly gendered and one that places the burden of infant morbidity and racial disparity on women themselves.

If only women had better intentions, the model intimates, outcomes would be better. The reproductive life plan is a tool that produces knowledge and produces social order.[77] It is a device used by clinicians to learn about and track reproductive desires, and it is a tool that is intended to organize how women should and do think about themselves, their reproductive futures, and their place in society. Moreover, reproductive life plans appeal to a sense of morality, motherhood, and individual responsibility among women who are not yet pregnant. Generalized health is the new—and gendered—morality.[78]

Further, this neoliberal ethos has been taken to the market: women are getting advice from magazines to take control and see their doctor, and they are increasingly faced with the prospect of "shopping their way" to reproductive safety through the practice of what sociologist Norah MacKendrick calls "precautionary consumption."[79] By priming and marketing the zero trimester to every woman, pre-pregnancy care positions reproductive responsibility squarely on the woman, her body, her life. Thus, the potentially pregnant period—the zero trimester—has become one with a neoliberal and consumerist overlay. Pre-pregnancy health discourse promotes the anticipation of motherhood and promulgates the idea that population health risk can be addressed through individual women's bodies and behaviors.[80] Scholars have highlighted how motherhood today is marked in large measure by consumption practices, with good motherhood tied to being able to buy children all the "things"—be they toys or healthy foods—that signal caring and meaning-making in a capitalist society. This consumer code extends not only to children but also to fetuses, through the rituals of baby showers and the planning of nurseries.

And it doesn't stop there. The *future fetus* is now an object of consumer culture. The pre-pregnancy care model pronounces that to engage in the healthiest pregnancy possible, women should plan well ahead, have an identifiable reproductive life plan, and buy advice books and products that will position them in the "responsible" category. Consumer culture no doubt targets maternal love and motherhood; the very "materiality of things (both made and mass-produced) is inseparable from the politics of mothering and the construction of mothers and babies as social beings" in our society.[81] The pre-pregnancy care approach has initiated a health and consumer culture aimed at the pre-maternal—at anticipatory mother-hood. Yet, women are not all treated the same way in the promotion of this public-health project. Women now are urged to engage and cultivate—through their health, behavioral, and consumer practices—a symbolic future baby love. Chapter 6 delves into how ideas about race, gender, risk, and maternity have shaped public-health promotion campaigns that ask women to do just that.

6 Promoting Maternal Visions

GENDER, RACE, AND FUTURE BABY LOVE

On Valentine's Day 2013, when many young women across the United States were attending performances of the "Vagina Monologues," having a romantic evening with their partner, or eschewing the commercial holiday altogether, the CDC launched a public health campaign aimed at getting young women to think about their future babies. Slated to run through Mother's Day of the same year, the "Show Your Love" campaign touted the importance of women's health prior to pregnancy. According to a press release, the campaign's message declared that a woman who wants to have a baby can "show love" for her nonexistent child through "first loving herself by adopting healthy habits well before becoming pregnant." The reward for women heeding this advice? "Your baby will thank you for it." Further, "living a healthy lifestyle is a way to show love to yourself and your future baby, long before a baby is in the plans."[1]

Chapter 5 focused on clinical and cultural uptake of the pre-pregnancy care model, and this chapter examines a specific example of how the model has been represented in public health promotion. The "Show Your Love" campaign materialized at an interesting juncture in the trajectory of the pre-pregnancy care model. As mentioned in previous chapters, public health advocates are not unaware of the criticisms directed at the pre-pregnancy care model as one that treats women as simply reproductive vessels. Given the feminist and popular critiques, one prominent pre-conception health expert wrote in 2010 that, for the agenda to be successful among all reproductive-aged women, the framework must work to include and recognize women who might not value motherhood in their near future (or ever).[2] The "Show Your Love" campaign of 2013 debuted after these appraisals, and the campaign materials were divided so as to create two separate target audiences: women who desire a future pregnancy and women who do not envision motherhood in their life plans.[3] The new campaign even drew on feminist rhetoric, professing that, "for those women who don't want to start a family in the near future or at all, the campaign encourages them to choose healthy behaviors so that they can be their best and achieve the goals and dreams they have set for themselves."[4]

Thus, the CDC's "Show Your Love" campaign represents a potent crystallization of the cultural and health trend toward reframing women in the name of pregnancy. This chapter shows that—notwithstanding recent shifts in strategy—CDC campaign rhetoric still positions all women of childbearing age as future mothers. According to these messages, women planning to get pregnant and those who are not planning to do so are equally potentially pregnant. I contend that the campaign serves as an example of public health authorities advocating for women to view themselves as potentially pregnant, in an attempt to shift the meaning of contemporary motherhood and womanhood to encompass the embodiment of a pre-maternal state. In giving a critical reading of the first release of the "Show Your Love" campaign as it materialized in 2013 (there have since been calls within the CDC's Preconception Health and Health Care Initiative to expand and diversify the campaign's message), I also highlight its feminized and racialized depictions of reproductive responsibility among women of childbearing age.

To analyze the manifestation of the pre-pregnancy care model in public health promotion, I looked to the materials produced by the CDC's "Show Your Love" campaign. According to the initial campaign materials, numerous national and state organizations have assisted in implementing the message, including the March of Dimes; the National Healthy Start Association;

Planned Parenthood Federation of America; and the Association of Women's Health, Obstetric and Neonatal Nurses. Thus, the CDC provided the raw materials for a nationwide campaign that was distributed not only through the CDC's official website but through numerous partner organizations. Partner organizations could link to the CDC's site, post educational videos and posters on their websites, and distribute materials directly to women. I studied the campaign site, including all of the "Show Your Love" materials produced by the CDC in the first installation of the campaign.[5] These materials were comprised of two logo images; two health checklists; two press releases; a list of partner organization talking points; fourteen posters; two public service announcement videos; four radio scripts; four podcast transcripts; four educational videos; three e-cards; and six image libraries with a total of 125 stock images, divided into the categories "Women Who Want to Become Pregnant" (n=33), "Women Who Do Not Want to Become Pregnant" (n=53), "Hugging" (n=7), "Nutrition" (n=12), "Physical Activity" (n=11), and "Visiting the Doctor" (n =9), intended for use by partner organizations to create their own materials.

Conducting textual analysis on these primary extant texts, I subjected the scripts to analytic scrutiny, paying close attention to the use of language, rhetoric, context, and emergent themes across the materials,[6] especially pertaining to maternal love, reproductive responsibility, risk temporality, and selfhood. Because most of the materials were packaged in the predetermined categories of "women who want to become pregnant" and "women who do not want to become pregnant," I documented differences in discursive strategy and imagery across target groups. Following other scholars who have studied campaigns that spotlight reproductive risk,[7] I focused on the "Show Your Love" campaign's discursive framework and how it developed and disseminated ideas about gender and health. There are limitations to studying the text and discourse of one public health initiative, to be sure, but the "Show Your Love" campaign constituted a deliberate nationwide attempt to shift thinking and practices around pre-pregnancy care. The CDC's "Show Your Love" campaign thus represents a bounded but powerful example not only of how maternal responsibility and selfhood are portrayed in public-health promotion today but also of how these meanings are being stretched to encompass more of a woman's life.

PUBLIC HEALTH AND SOCIAL CONTROL

Scholars have documented how public-health promotion can hype health risks[8] and function as an agent of social control.[9] Health promotion often is bound up in a pursuit of moral virtue,[10] and public-health policies promote health as a "moral imperative."[11] Over the course of the twentieth century, medicine and public health increasingly converged on emphasizing individual risk factors as explanations for disease, even as, at the same time, diseases shifted away from the infectious and toward the chronic—that is, toward diseases that usually are multi-causal.[12] Moreover, sociologist Sarah Nettleton wrote in the 1990s that we were witnessing "a new paradigm of health and medicine," a "psycho-social-environmental/epidemiological model and the appearance of a long overdue commitment to the prevention of disease."[13] Nettleton argues that the new ideological assumptions that accompany this shift are predicated on "risk, surveillance, and the rational self," which often assist "prevailing sexist assumptions" that shape public-health promotion and policy.[14] This shift also highlights individual behavior at the same time that it intensifies population surveillance of health. As Brandt and Rozin write, "Increasingly, we are told that new knowledge gives us new opportunities to take control of our health."[15]

When this control imperative is compounded with the moral necessity to provide the best health for a future baby, the ontological burden of reproductive outcomes potentially shifts for women. Women's rights are then perhaps ignored; public-health officials have averred, at various points in American history, that securing the public's health occasionally must be accomplished at the expense of individual rights.[16] In cases of pregnancy health, it is usually women's rights that are at stake. Public health discourse in particular has been mined as a fruitful arena in which to examine the relationship among women's rights, authoritative knowledge, representations of fetuses, and reproductive bodies.[17] Feminist scholars increasingly have also noted the expansion of pregnancy and public health discourse aimed at women not visibly pregnant and even at those who are not pregnant at all, discourse that treats all women of reproductive age as if they should be primed for pregnancy.[18]

I show that what is stressed in the CDC's "Show Your Love" campaign is that expected motherhood is assumed to be embodied, not only as something that can be practiced through social activities or healthy behaviors but also as something to be internalized vis-à-vis the commanding messages of institutions that disperse medical and public health recommendations. The campaign's message touted self-love and baby love simultaneously, conflating womanhood and motherhood. The "Show Your Love" campaign built on previous tropes of maternal love, devotion, and sacrifice. While this trend is clearly established in feminist critiques of health recommendations to women, by focusing these concepts on non-pregnant women, this campaign introduced a new ideal form of the contemporary reproductive life experience.

My analysis of the "Show Your Love" campaign begins by showing that not only were all women of reproductive age positioned as future mothers but that the campaign also employed a novel, future-oriented gift rhetoric, charging women with the responsibility of showing affection ("show your love") to future babies through current material behaviors. The promise of the message was that women will receive babies' gratitude in return. I argue that the discourse of the "Show Your Love" campaign thus cultivated an ethic of anticipatory motherhood and a pre-maternal selfhood, exhorting non-pregnant women to act on their present selves to provide for a future other. Within this overarching narrative, I also discuss evidence of racialized distinctions around reproductive intentionality, with white women depicted as "planners" and women of color as "non-planners." I argue that, while it tried to appease feminist critics by incorporating women who are not thinking about motherhood as a master status, the campaign reified dominant tropes about women as mothers and about the types of women who exhibit reproductive responsibility. I end by discussing the potential implications of the "Show Your Love" campaign for current feminist debates about motherhood in the public sphere.

ROMANCING THE FUTURE

How are women to show their prospective maternal love? One "Show Your Love" campaign video ran in reverse chronological order, beginning with a white woman cuddling a baby. A voice declared, "Showing your love doesn't start here." The next scene revealed the woman holding her pregnant belly, drinking a bottle of water, with the narration, "Showing your love doesn't start here." Then the voice repeated, "Showing your love doesn't start here," revealing a bottle of wine being replaced by a bottle of water in the woman's refrigerator. The narrator explained, "Showing your love begins before you get pregnant. . . . Loving your baby starts with your preconception health."[19] By defining pre-conception health behaviors as expressions of maternal love, the video imposed an embodied and inter-twined sense of morality, motherhood, and individual responsibility among women who are not yet pregnant.

This futuristic rhetoric permeated the wide variety of pre-pregnancy planning materials produced by the CDC. At the beginning of one radio piece intended for women planning a pregnancy, a woman is heard (who according to the script is in her thirties) saying, "You've been dreaming of showing a baby all your love in the future. But you don't need to wait to show your love! Loving your baby starts with preconception health." The script then listed healthy behaviors and stated, amid the sounds of an infant in the background, that pre-pregnancy health is important "because healthy women make healthier mothers, and healthy mothers make healthier babies." The target woman was directed to the CDC's website to "learn how to get your body ready for pregnancy," ending with "your baby will thank you for it!" The strategy here motivated the listener by "remind-ing" her that she has been dreaming of loving a baby—intimating that maternal thinking suffuses women's intellectual energies. Indeed, mater-nal affection can begin now, through attention to pre-pregnancy health.

By recommending that women ready their bodies for inevitable babies, the "Show Your Love" campaign drew on the modern idea of the planning project of the self—just as the reproductive life plans did (as shown in Chapter 5)—while at the same time highlighting the paradox between a population-level project and the individualized subject of the discourse.[20] Michel Foucault writes that technologies of the self enable individuals to impact the way they are in the world "so as to transform themselves in order to attain a certain state of happiness, purity, wisdom, perfection, or immortality."[21] If a healthy future baby is happiness and perfection, then women's current selves are likely to adhere to and internalize changes that will affect this outcome. In this vein, pre-pregnancy discourse exploits the experience of the "risk society," in which we are oriented toward taming the future through current practices.[22] In essence, the modern sense of ontological security and anxiety obliges individuals "to think ahead, to anticipate future possibilities," even amid the inability to perfectly control potential outcomes.[23] Although child health ultimately is uncontrollable, pre-pregnancy risk messages mix this uncertainty with discourse touting the ability to control one's body and the health outcomes of others in the contemporary reproductive landscape.[24]

Indeed, these CDC recommendations fit cultural trends mentioned throughout this book—especially toward treating the (risky) future, or simply life itself, through the present by engaging in anticipatory social and material practices aimed at optimizing one's health.[25] Self-discipline discourse vis-à-vis reproductive risk is undeniably amplified and extended with the "Show Your Love" campaign, as the message revolved around fetuses that are assumed to be conceived in the future. Social surveillance, appraisal, and advice regarding fetal risks are no longer situated on a gestating woman but simply on a woman of reproductive age. All young women were presented in this campaign as containing the potentiality of future life, shifting the ontology of maternity to the pre-pregnant body. For example, women today prepare their pre-maternal bodies by eating organic foods or avoiding tuna as a kind of future-oriented behavior of risk reduction.[26] Rather than understanding reproductive risk as something located in broader society, these precautionary practices ultimately fall on individual women and their day-to-day behaviors.[27]

This kind of self-disciplining behavior, and thus the sharpening of the pre-maternal self, was operationalized and promoted in the "Show Your Love" campaign materials through health checklists on the campaign website. Two different checklists detailed goals for improving the lifestyle of women with seemingly different ideas about their goals for motherhood. Both documents listed behavior regulations such as eating healthy foods, staying active, making sure vaccinations are up to date, and reducing alcohol intake. The checklist labeled for "planners" was clearly focused on a future baby—"Show Your LOVE! Steps to a Healthier Me and Baby-to-Be!"[28]—but the checklist for "non-planners" made more covert references to the future baby. Although the title emphasized only a "Healthier Me,"[29] the checklist included items directed toward improving pre-pregnancy health. For example, it indicated that taking folic acid daily "will help prevent birth defects of the brain and spine should I decide to or accidentally get pregnant."[30] The materials betrayed how contingent pregnancy is—presenting it as an ever-present possibility and assuming that an unintended pregnancy will proceed to birth.[31] The checklist cautioned at the end, "remember that life happens, and plans can change."

Although both lists recognized the flexibility of sticking with goals, the "non-planner" document also indicated that "if you decide you want to have a baby sometime in the near future, be sure to plan your pregnancy and get your body ready before you get pregnant!" Evident here again was a valorization of the planned approach to health, tacking onto our cultural preoccupation with neoliberal personal responsibility and calculated life choices that emerged in the last chapter.[32] To find ontological security in womanhood and in maternity, every individual woman, according to the "Show Your Love" campaign, must anticipate any possibility of pregnancy and any potential risks to the health of that pregnancy. For women of reproductive age, the ethic of anticipatory motherhood dictates that the future self is understood as a maternal self. Womanhood is now represented in a framework of the maternal future.

BUILDING PRE-MATERNAL DEVOTION

What is a woman to do to cultivate her maternal future? The text of a poster (*see* Figure 5) intended for women thinking about getting pregnant explained that "it's time to nurture and love yourself by planning and preparing your body for pregnancy." The poster invited women to "choose behaviors like eating a healthy diet," "stop drinking alcohol," and speak with a physician "about how to best manage" medical concerns and conditions "with pregnancy in mind." The poster ended with the tagline "Your Baby Will Thank You for It!" This message is couched in terms of self-care, but the end goal remained the elicitation of a future baby's gratitude.[33]

The glorification of anticipatory motherhood and the plea for an empathic self-love (a form of future-love), rather than love for a real baby, draws on gendered ways of thinking about styles of love, with women associated with emotive love and men with physical love.[34] Additionally, the call to produce love for babies—abstractly and in advance—creates an

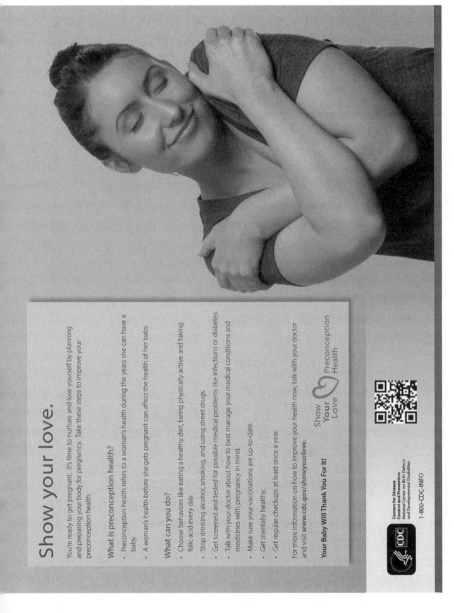

Figure 5. "Show Your Love" campaign poster produced by the National Center on Birth Defects and Developmental Disabilities of the Centers for Disease Control and Prevention, 2013. Targeted toward women planning to get pregnant, this poster lists specific steps women can take to improve their health before becoming pregnant. (© 2013 the Centers for Disease Control and Prevention; reprinted with permission; color version available online)

affective relationship between the woman and the nonexistent baby. The idea is that she provides a pre-prepared healthy womb, and the baby, when present, will thank her for it. This is a literal, rather than simply symbolic construction of gift giving, as the gift of love here is indeed part of the giver—it is derived from the woman's body (from her self-love), which builds the affective bond. The "Show Your Love" discourse was predicated on the idea that the woman ostensibly will be thanked later for supplying this gift, conjuring up the social expectation that mothers (but, here, women more broadly) are expected to do things selflessly, sacrificing without the expectation of return. This tactic was a crafty way of saying that self-care and self-love have utility—that, in a way, selfishness is acceptable if it helps to improve the health of others. Self-love, then, is only understood within the discourse of anticipatory motherhood. Self-love becomes a form of self-sacrifice. Because babies—or children, for that matter—do not usually express gratitude for being healthy or for being raised, the sacrifice can be seen as part of an unreciprocated gift. The self-love in actuality could function as a perfunctory endeavor, one that draws on rhetoric of generosity and gratitude. By urging women to care about their selves through a lens of anticipatory motherhood, the campaign extended the ethos of maternal self-sacrifice long before a pregnancy is achieved.

Feminist scholars have theorized about the corporeal aspects of maternal generosity, embodied gifts, and bodily sacrifice. Pregnancy, breastfeeding, and gamete donation, for instance, all involve the process of giving part of one's self to another.[35] In the case of surrogate motherhood, for example, wherein women can experience an ontological divide between current self and future self vis-à-vis their reproductive endeavors, surrogates have been found to engage in love and gifting rhetoric to make sense of their complicated and commodified "journey."[36] By contrast, or perhaps by extension, the "Show Your Love" campaign deployed a future-oriented corporeal generosity, asking all reproductive-capable women to be healthy now so that they can give their future babies the gift of life and health.

Perhaps to downplay the potential burden imposed by an ethic of anticipatory motherhood, the campaign drew on a feminist discourse of choice and independence that highlights women's social and economic achievements. For example, a "non-planner" public-service announcement script described three women: one in her late teens, one in her mid-twenties, one in her thirties. The teen wondered aloud if she should get her degree, while the woman in her thirties explained that women's futures are bright. The sound effect in the background, as dictated by the script, was the "soft cooing of a baby when she mentions different paths." This approach undermined the point of the "planning" distinction among women, inserting baby sounds to point women to what they really want. The campaign's pre-pregnancy rhetoric was organized around a sense of empowerment, yet it is one that undercut any path other than the one to motherhood. Following is the text from another written transcript (in which the age of the sole narrator is stipulated):

> (Woman in mid 20s): Women have more opportunities today than ever before. Do I want to get my degree, start my career, travel? The different paths are endless . . . and while I do want a family someday, a baby is not in my plan right now.
>
> The different paths open to women today are endless. Becoming as healthy as possible will help me on ANY path I choose. So join me by starting today and show yourself some love! Take time to improve your physical and mental health now. Eat a healthy diet, be physically active, and see your doctor at least once a year. . . and if you are having sex and a baby is not part of your plan right now, use an effective method of contraception correctly and consistently . . . just like I do.
>
> Stop drinking excessive amounts of alcohol and don't smoke or use street drugs.
>
> School, career, travel, family. . . . To be ready for any path you choose, start making healthy choices today. Show your love to the most important person in the world—you! Visit www.cdc.gov/showyourlove[37]

The furtive marketing move in this radio piece was to position "preconception health" as "women's health," while in fact the focus was still on the future baby. In appealing to the opportunities young women have today as a result of feminist advances—"the different paths are endless"—there is a concurrent and subtle assumption that the listener probably desires "a family someday." To be ready for any path is to be ready for a future baby, as women were directed to the CDC's pre-conception health website, a site that presented a framework that clearly positioned health in terms of reproductive status.

This characterization matters for the contemporary young women's subjectivity and experiences. For instance, in one educational video aimed at "non-planners," a young black woman explained her plan for her job, career, and ideal lifestyle. The very fact that she was planning her life but labeled a "non-planner," because she was not immediately hoping to have a baby, reveals that reproductive planning is considered the most valued form of planning in this pre-pregnancy framework. The supplied text that accompanied this particular video explains: "Right now, you're looking out for you—and that's a good thing. Your health is really important to help you achieve your goals and fulfill your dreams. Find out how to take care of yourself now—and for the 'you' of the future." The "you" in the final phrase here was inexplicably set in quotation marks. The "you" of the future most likely includes motherhood. When women are "non-planners," the "you" can genuinely stand in for "you," but once a woman starts planning a pregnancy or becomes pregnant, as the other videos and scripts in this analysis indicate, the "you" is subsumed by a future baby.

DEMARCATING THE PRE-PREGNANT POPULATION

Who is and isn't recognized in the pre-pregnant population? Although the press release for the "Show Your Love" campaign indicated that "preconception health is the health of women and men during their reproductive years," the overwhelming target of the campaign materials was women, once again. The pre-conception phase is before pregnancy, and one might envision men and women being treated equally since they contribute equally to the future conception.[38] Yet the campaign was manifestly gendered, as it was all about women in their childbearing years. Indeed, the line about the health of women and men from the press release was directly followed by this sentence: "Preconception health focuses on women taking important steps now to protect their health and the health of the family they may want to have sometime in the future." Men were swiftly taken out of the picture.

Furthermore, there was no discernible attempt to capture diversity in maternal intention status beyond "planners" versus "non-planners"—for instance, lesbian women did not appear, nor did women who *never* want to have children. Although the campaign nominally included women "who cannot have children" as part of its category of "currently not planning," there was no mention of adoption or surrogacy or any arrangement in which the body and the maternal do not align in practice.

Additionally, my reading shows that the campaign gestured toward racialized representations of the types of women who plan pregnancies and those who do not. For example, the campaign materials that were labeled for "planners" included all white, light-skinned women and heterosexual couples. When this analysis was undertaken in April 2013, soon after the launch of the campaign, I found that out of thirty-three images in the "planners" image library (comprised of stock images for use by partner organizations to create their own materials), not one woman was dark-skinned. At that time, the campaign's fifty-three images in the library targeting "non-planners" were by contrast made up entirely of what appear to be African American and Latina women, and no one in this particular library was represented as part of a romantic partnership. Only one image of a light-skinned woman overlapped both libraries. This stark racial divide continued with respect to the published posters targeting women who want to become pregnant (all women pictured were light-skinned) and the posters for women who do not want to become pregnant (the main focus of these posters was a dark-skinned woman). Although partner organizations presumably could use these images to accompany any message, the racial divide in the initial categorization was striking.

The rest of this section focuses on three videos released by the 2013 campaign that depicted different racial groups.[39] My observations of racialization come from evidence mostly in the form of images, rather than only in prose, and I point out that these observations, while incipient, might have significant implications for reproductive-risk discourse.

One video featured a white man and woman, one featured a young African American woman, and one featured a Latina mother. The first video, for "planners" and labeled "couple," follows a white heterosexual couple in exercise clothes walking outdoors. The woman begins by saying, "Me? Have a baby? We're thinking about it, in the next year or so." The woman explains that they told their doctor about their plans, who in turn told them about the importance of pre-conception health. At this point in the video, the man stops, throws open his arms in confusion, says "Pre-what?" and laughs. The woman also laughs, grabs his arm, and explains that pre-conception health can affect the health of their baby. The man nods and says, "Well, that caught our attention." The woman then lists all the things she needs to do: take a multivitamin, get physically active, and so on. As is seen in other materials, the same themes were presented in this video. While the couple indicated that they are "in this together," the attention was on the woman's behavior, aided by her partner's moral support. They said they are exercising to improve their pre-conception health. The implication was that any current healthy behaviors are not intended merely for their individual health but for the health of any future baby, thereby giving the abstract gift of future love. The couple wrapped up the video by saying that they still have a lot of planning ahead of them and that at least now they know about pre-conception health and why it's essential for "our baby-to-be."

Embedded in this script was a concerted sense of guarding against risk through planning that is followed by an exhibition of relief that they are now on the prescribed path. Represented was a white, heterosexual couple who have ostensibly done what they are supposed to do. They have seen their doctor, are responsibly controlling their reproductive lives, have received health advice prior to pregnancy, and are now implementing pre-pregnancy recommendations in their daily life.

The setup of the second video was quite different; this file was labeled "Jada" and featured a young, apparently single, African American woman. The script starts with Jada saying, "Me, have a baby? Are you kidding? I work a part-time job and I'm getting ready to go to college to be a nurse. I'll choose when I want to start a family; until then, I'm gonna stay on my birth control pills. I wanna do well in school to get a good job, so, I'm taking care of my health." She explains that she learned from her doctor to take a multivitamin to get the folic acid she needs. Ostensibly this action is for a future baby, even though Jada indicates that she does not want a baby in the near future. The video ended with the recommendation to "Show yourself some love. There are important things that you can do for you. Set your goals and make a plan today."

There is feminist utility in presenting young women with multiple life choices, and there is certainly more than a glint of empowerment discourse here. Yet, there is also a class- and age-based undercurrent in the depiction of Jada as a promising young woman in a financially unstable position, as she works part-time while studying to be a nurse. Furthermore, the video called to mind stereotypical ideas about black single motherhood and the corresponding cultural notion that black men are not reliable co-parents.[40] Jada was unpartnered in the video, and her script emphasized self-reliance. When compared to the video of the white couple, the implication in this video is that black women must hone self-sufficiency—a theme that overlaps with cultural stereotypes of the strong black woman who is ultimately alone in planning her future.[41] Indeed, in this video, the singular pronoun "I" was invoked by Jada, as contrasted with the use of "we" and "our" by the white couple.

The third video was labeled "Maria" and featured a Latina mother. Similar to the "Jada" video described above, the fact that this mother was depicted as alone with a toddler suggests that the father is not as directly involved in his child's care. This might indirectly reproduce stereotypes about Latino men as absent fathers as well. The video starts off with Maria saying, "Me have another baby? No estoy lista!—I'm not ready!" She explains that she has her "hands full" with her baby daughter Rosa. Her doctor has told her not to smoke or use illegal drugs and not to have more than one alcoholic drink a day. She explains, "But I know that when we start trying to get pregnant again, I can't drink anything with alcohol in it at all." Moreover, Maria has diabetes, and she says that "if I don't keep my blood sugar in control it can affect my health and the health of my next baby. So, I make regular doctor visits so that I keep a close watch on that. Rosa gets her vaccinations, and so do I! I want to be as healthy as I can so that I can keep up with this little one." She ends with the proclamation that pre-conception health is important "for you and your family." In this script, there are calls to show love to oneself, to the current baby, to the future baby, and to the family, which positions the Latina mother as the embodiment of domestic care.

The covers of the videos and corresponding e-cards on the campaign site showed the white couple actively planning with a doctor, Jada by herself, and Maria with her child. Each depicted scenario drew upon cultural stereotypes of gender, race, and reproductive health. The white couple is presented as responsible planners. The young African American woman is shown to be single and working while going to school. The Latina mother is revealed to have diabetes, and her partner, Juan, is mentioned although not present in the video.

That the campaign released three videos—with women of different ethnic backgrounds represented in each—underlines the differential ways in which pre-pregnancy health is marketed to target population groups, reflecting racialized tropes used in health promotion. Popular representations of reproduction often not only are racialized but also are stratified by class and national origin, and these depictions have continued in the twenty-first century.[42] Feminist scholars have long documented how women of different racial categories are treated differently in discourse and in public policy regarding reproduction as well as in the U.S. health care system more broadly.[43] The illustrative term in the social sciences is stratified reproduction.

First coined by Shellee Colen,[44] stratified reproduction refers to the differential experience, value, and reward of reproductive labor "according to inequalities of access to material and social resources in particular historical and cultural contexts." The term aptly describes the "power relations by which some categories of people are empowered to nurture and reproduce, while others are disempowered."[45] Black womanhood in particular historically has been, and continues to be, beset by fraught symbols of sexual and maternal politics.[46] As Dorothy Roberts's work so eloquently emphasizes, it is not only the sexist aspects of reproductive imagery and discourse that we must contend with as feminist scholars but also the racist standards that inhere in this arena as well.[47] Indeed, reproductive discourse in America does not just involve gender politics; it is also a discourse of racial politics. What it means to be defined as a good or a bad mother has persistent racial undertones.[48] The "Show Your Love" campaign highlights the stubborn sexist and racialized notions of anticipatory motherhood.

It is worth noting that, as part of a public health campaign, these racialized images are likely intended to reflect public-health demographics. As has been mentioned in previous chapters, black women, for instance, are more likely than other women to experience adverse birth outcomes or unintended pregnancies.[49] Black and Hispanic children have a greater likelihood of living apart from their fathers than do white children.[50] Immigrant Latinas are known to have a prenatal advantage over native Latinas (known as the "Latina paradox"); despite this reality, as Alyshia Gálvez has shown in her study,[51] health care providers often continue to reinforce racialized stereotypes in reproductive care. Racism has a profound impact on health outcomes, as does the category of race as a social construct.[52]

When public-health messages try to reflect demographics and at-risk groups, they in effect produce powerful symbols that reproduce stereotypes and ignore the systematic inequalities that inform the demographic realities regarding health disparities in the United States. Even if the campaign creators perceived these images as part of a pragmatic approach to health promotion, the language and representation in these texts and images matter.

Constructed self-love and baby love were presented in the campaign materials as forms of affection that are set up to reflect which women "should" be paying more attention to themselves or to their potential fetuses. The "Show Your Love" public-health campaign attempted a subtle discursive move, one that situates responsible "planners"—or the ones who intimate that they want a baby soon—as white heterosexual women and thus the "good" population of potentially pregnant women. As Linda Blum's work reveals, social or public health discourse that might be leveraged to laud white women at the same time could be used to debase black women.[53] This campaign's rhetoric perpetuates the idea that women of color need to be told to plan their fertility, use contraception, and change their behaviors, and white women are situated as model citizens, ready to hone their future baby love. This discursive arrangement reveals how women of color continue to be on the margins of "good" motherhood.

CULTIVATING THE MATERNAL FUTURE

The CDC's "Show Your Love" campaign is an illustrative example not only of how maternal responsibility is portrayed in contemporary public health promotion but also how it is being stretched to encompass more of a woman's life. Women were linked to a romanticized maternal future through this campaign, one that pivots on a fresh form of future-oriented devotion. Promoting moral motherhood and maternal love through social and health practices is not new, but much of this endeavor has previously focused on pregnant women or mothers. Pregnancy, for instance, is an obvious visual depiction of the fertile body, a body that tempts monitoring by society and experts.[54]

In nineteenth-century America, the selflessness and sacrifice of motherhood was given a central part in building the moral character of children and the state; as Jan Lewis shows,[55] a woman was to exhibit self-love and self-control ("her most strenuous efforts would have to be directed at herself") so that her children would someday embody their mother's love. Starting in the Progressive Era, women in the United States were called upon to obtain expert advice from medical and public health practitioners about how best to raise children, resulting in what Rima Apple calls "scientific motherhood,"[56] essentially medicalizing and moralizing motherhood.[57] By the end of the twentieth century, the ideology of intensive mothering[58]—the labor-intensive, expert-driven, emotionally consuming, and child-centered mode of contemporary motherhood in the United States—helped to explain the persistence of maternal sacrifice. This concept sensitized Joan Wolf's twenty-first-century characterization of maternal sacrifice, "total motherhood," which accents the idea that mothers are exhorted to "devote themselves wholly to reducing risks to their children" throughout their reproductive life course.[59] And the idea of maternal sacrifice remains "central to the ways in which normative ideas about motherhood are constructed and understood."[60] Public health promotion has functioned to promote future maternal love and sacrifice, thus also encouraging a novel kind of social control over women's behaviors and bodies.

Yet these previous analyses focused mostly on risk messages directed at women who are already mothers. Intensive mothering and total motherhood extended backward in the "Show Your Love" materials to focus more exclusively on the pre-maternal self, to what I have called in this book "anticipatory motherhood"—a framework that situates all women of childbearing age as ontologically pre-pregnant. Women have long been positioned as the responsible party for the health of a fetus, but with the ethic of anticipatory motherhood, women now also are positioned as the vector for any outcomes of a future fetus. Indeed, in these materials the importance of a woman's self is positioned as contingent on her maternal future. Although a woman's self is inevitably fluid throughout the life course (regardless of whether she decides to have children), a woman's self-meaning in her reproductive years becomes understood in terms of a pre-maternal state, thereby foregrounding the reproductive self above and beyond any other form of selfhood.

It makes sense for women (and men) to lead healthy lives and care about their reproductive plans, and it is a feminist platform to focus on planning and life choices when it comes to reproduction. But what does it mean for how we view women's roles in society when womanhood is couched in terms of anticipatory motherhood? Defining women primarily as reproductive vessels is anathema to women's rights discourses. By advocating women's health in terms of providing love for unconceived babies, this campaign set us back several decades in essentially defining all women of reproductive age first and foremost as pre-pregnant bodies—women not yet pregnant, women who likely have not thought of pregnancy or, if they have, have not yet internalized the responsibility of potential guilt associated with pre-pregnancy discourse.

Due to critiques of pre-pregnancy health promotion prior to this campaign, there was a marked discourse in the "Show Your Love" materials of love for future baby and love for self. The campaign also attempted to distinguish between women who are planning pregnancies and women who are not. The "non-planner," though, is of course an oxymoron—an attempt to appease feminist critics that devolves into normative notions of proper and improper maternal behavior. The message is that good motherhood and bad motherhood can be inscribed by the behaviors of all female bodies. As the campaign attempted to distinguish women's desires—acceding that some women do not want a pregnancy in the near future or even at all—it reinforced the dominant trope that women of childbearing age are mothers-in-waiting, solely responsible for reproductive outcomes.

This focus on planning for future babies was also positioned racially in the "Show Your Love" materials. Defining appropriate future baby love as something that is not only gendered and heteronormative but also something that is stratified based on race furthers racist cultural projections of women of color as unprepared to exhibit reproductive responsibility, placing these women in a riskier category within the potentially pregnant population. By differentiating the potentially pregnant based on intentionality—those women who are planning to have a baby in the near future and those who are not—we see the burnishing of racially stratified undertones around pregnancy intentions.

This analysis of the dissemination of pre-pregnancy messages begs the question: What happens if the ethic of anticipatory motherhood permeates policy? Does this discursive stratification of the maternal future matter for lived reality? The campaign sentiment of love and gratitude, as seen in these health-promotion materials, can theoretically be extended: If a woman can be thanked for heeding pre-pregnancy health recommendations, then she can also be held accountable for not holding to them. We have to then worry about the possible criminalization of potentially pregnant women. Lynn Paltrow and Jeanne Flavin in their rigorous examination of coercive interventions on pregnant women in the United States post–*Roe v. Wade*, find that "pregnant African American women are significantly more likely to be arrested, reported by hospital staff, and subjected to felony charges" in issues of drug use, for example.[61] Criminalizing women for prenatal behaviors (e.g., the crack baby "epidemic") could conceivably be extended to all reproductive-aged women, but especially minority women, in the pre-pregnancy era.[62]

Feminist intellectuals such as Elisabeth Badinter have argued that it is counterproductive for contemporary women to spend so much time and energy on quotidian mothering tasks like breast-feeding or washing cloth diapers.[63] This has been a source of heated debate in the public arena. But what if we take a further step back, before pregnancy and motherhood occur, and consider what an ethic of anticipatory motherhood would do to contemporary womanhood among those of reproductive age? What if all young women internalize this rhetoric and in good faith treat their everyday bodies as pre-pregnant in the name of a future fetus? What consequences would this have for women's status and subjectivity in society? If this discourse takes hold in contemporary society, it could be an unfamiliar world, with the potentially pregnant population heeding pre-pregnancy health advice and acting out a pre-maternal selfhood. Or, perhaps women would feel empowered by this planning-for-the-future discourse, seeing their bodies as the ultimate and powerful convergence of health, self, and family future. As motherhood studies continue to fill a rich area for feminist scholarship, we should pay close and critical attention to the rise of anticipatory motherhood and caution against a worldview that envisions all women as pre-maternal, one in which women are charged with loving fetuses and babies that do not exist.

7 Governing Risk, Governing Women

ANTICIPATORY MOTHERHOOD AND SOCIAL ORDER

On May 8, 2013, at a meeting of the American College of Obstetricians and Gynecologists (ACOG) in New Orleans, Jeanne A. Conry began her presidential address by proclaiming: "This is the year of the woman. That's right. This is the year of the woman."[1] Conry—a renowned obstetrician-gynecologist who holds both a PhD and an MD—was onto something. The passage of health care reform under President Obama had initiated expansive policy recognition of the need for preventive women's health services, and she argued that in the United States "we have agreed that the health of women is a priority." Conry's remarks focused, in part, on improving pre-pregnancy care, arguing that women need to be healthy across their life course. The title of her speech—"Every Woman, Every Time"—was a clear homage to the mantra of the pre-pregnancy care model as advocated by CDC experts. Conry, in fact, served as chair of the California Preconception Care Council prior to assuming leadership of ACOG. That she used her presidential address to highlight the importance of pre-pregnancy care reflected just how far the idea had come.

We are today hyper-vigilant about the reproductive potential of women of childbearing age. Health promotion messages and physician recommendations abound, urging women to take care of themselves in the service of future reproduction. This enhanced attentiveness to the pre-pregnancy period is not just top-down. At a time when women, on average, are having fewer babies and having them later in life, individuals buy pre-pregnancy health books to increase their chances of healthy conceptions. Some professional women freeze their eggs while pursuing their career, to ensure the possibility of future biological parenthood and to avoid the risks of later childbearing. The boundaries of reproductive risk shifted at the turn of the twenty-first century to highlight pre-pregnancy risk factors and to frame maternal duties as beginning before pregnancy. As we increasingly attempt to tame risk in all its realities and potentialities, we must also be attuned to how risk messages impact the way we think about, internalize, and broadly understand the material situation of individuals in society. In care related to pregnancy, especially, medical ideas intersect with social policy to change the lived realities of women.

This book has shown how broad-based ideas about pre-pregnancy behavior and intervention became possible—even popular—in the twenty-first century. In the first decade of this new century, pre-pregnancy care was not something of common knowledge, not in public dialogue nor among medical experts. Now it animates the thinking of women's health practitioners and policy makers nationwide. Ten years after the CDC launched its initiative for the cause, pre-pregnancy care has become a dominant and pervasive way to think about reproductive risk.

INSTITUTIONALIZING THE PRE-PREGNANCY FRAMEWORK

The advent of what I call "the zero trimester" reflects increasing attention being placed on pre-pregnancy care as the answer to better birth outcomes in America. Pre-pregnancy care emerged out of a moment of stalled progress, and amid a landscape of failed clinical intervention with prenatal care; indeed, the field of maternal and child health faced a conundrum at the end of the twentieth century. The prenatal care model—assumed to be the "magic bullet" for improving birth outcomes—was called into question by some obstetricians because, despite abundant expansions in service and coverage, it did not improve critical population health measures such as infant mortality. Obstetricians wrote with renewed urgency about the need to pull prenatal care backward—to expand it, not to eliminate it. Physicians and public-health experts essentially rediscovered the idea of pre-pregnancy care in the literature and, with a moral imperative, the CDC adopted the idea.

As is demonstrated throughout this book, pre-pregnancy care itself was not an entirely new idea. Physician accounts of women's pre-pregnancy health risks date back decades in medical journals; such concerns emerged especially during times when medical professionals expressed worries with the future of the race or with the social status of women. Of principal concern to maternal and child health experts at the turn of the twenty-first century were pregnancy intentions, with many pregnancies being categorized as mistimed or unwanted. It stood to reason that if women engaged in pre-pregnancy care and planned their pregnancies, then risk could be reduced. Yet, the experts who participated in defining and promoting the idea of pre-pregnancy care were hindered by an apparent dearth of evidence tying pre-pregnancy care to birth outcomes. To fill knowledge gaps, experts—including at the CDC—relied on reductionist cultural assumptions about women's maternal responsibilities and women's bodies as inherently reproductive. Thus, the rhetoric of pre-pregnancy care became quite controversial, as it seemingly validated anti-feminist notions of defining womanhood only in terms of motherhood or potential motherhood. To many people, this rhetoric was a backward and sexist attempt to frame women as nothing more than reproductive vessels.

However, existing assessments of the rise of the pre-pregnancy care framework have missed how a frame of reproductive justice helps to explain this shift in attention from prenatal to pre-pregnancy risk. Pre-pregnancy care was assumed by many experts to be an avenue for expanding women's reproductive autonomy, not limiting it. Pre-pregnancy care experts have long understood that women in the United States—especially low-income women—do not always have access to comprehensive health care across their life course, with one vital exception: when they are pregnant. The social policy trajectory in this country has been to value health coverage during pregnancy, with both private and public insurance plans allowing preventive health care coverage for women once a pregnancy is confirmed. In the U.S. social and political landscape, women's health has been valued mainly in the safe space of maternity. Experts realized that if women's health care could be defined in maternal terms— "pre-pregnancy"—then women might be able to receive comprehensive health care throughout their reproductive years. Although there increasingly are calls among researchers for gender inclusivity in pre-pregnancy care, men for the most part have been left out of this project altogether, despite also being potential reproducers.[2]

THE IMPACT OF REPRODUCTIVE SILOS

In discussing the contemporary backdrop of reproductive politics, experts with whom I spoke outlined clear strains in the reproductive arena that demarcated the reproductive silos of reproductive health care and maternal health care. As Chapter 4 detailed, many decades of policy making and social changes led to the starkly-felt division—even in the twenty-first century—between experts who focus on reproductive health care and those who focus on maternal health care. There is overlap between these worlds to be sure,[3] nevertheless the ideological and policy divisions were presented to me as deep and glaring: maternal health care is perceived to safeguard babies through pregnancy care, and reproductive health care is interested in pregnancy planning and spacing—in other words, its goal is to prevent babies. In the case of an unintended pregnancy, the reproductive silos are felt intensely. If a woman wants to continue her unintended pregnancy, she seeks maternity care; otherwise, she seeks reproductive care.

This dichotomized system has deep roots in the reproductive politics of America. The division of reproductive spheres, to some extent, stems from controversies over the legalization of abortion that led to family planning, contraception, and abortion care being separated from health care related to "wanted" pregnancies. I argue that this complicated history profoundly influenced the development and shape of the pre-pregnancy care model and the rise of the "zero trimester," as pre-pregnancy care advocacy in the twenty-first century began to try to blend these divisive realms. It seemed practical to maternal and child health care experts to use women's potential motherhood status to bridge the legacy of these distinct reproductive worlds and to offer an expanded frame of women's health. The pre-pregnancy care model, then, was in part intended as a political workaround to bring the two blocs of reproductive care and maternity care under the same umbrella, forming a "tacit coalition" without having to incorporate—formally, at least—politically contentious topics.[4]

The paradigmatic shift in thinking about pregnancy care, from the siloed-vision of prenatal care to the life-course approach of pre-pregnancy care, was meant to be a liberating force for women, removing the separation of maternal contingencies from their health care. To be sure, motherhood is no longer understood as the sole purpose of a woman's life, and women's reproductive health is generally viewed in a much more expansive frame than simply maternity care. Further, many women today are opting out of motherhood or seeking "alternative" avenues into maternity, such as through adoption or surrogacy. Moreover, as mentioned, age at first birth for women in America has increased steadily over the past several decades, and women are having fewer children than in the past.[5] A contemporary woman spends much of her reproductive life not pregnant—or, depending on one's preference, pre-pregnant.

Yet, to carve the maternal contingencies from comprehensive women's health care, experts used the strategy of maternalism when defining women as "potentially pregnant," a category that did not clearly fall in any previously defined reproductive worlds. The experts I interviewed were both acutely aware of the political realities that have unfairly tied women's health care to maternity *and* were quick to define women's health care in terms of maternity. In a way, pre-pregnancy care was positioned by experts not as a reductionist policy that views women as simply baby-making machines but as a resolutely progressive policy, as the best idea they had to address the entrenched reproductive care silos and the political firestorm of reproductive health in America. It was the very legacy of reproductive silos that allowed for pre-pregnancy care to emerge and be, at once, both highly controversial and highly agreeable.

PRE-PREGNANCY INTERVENTION AS "COMMON SENSE"

Of course, intention, dissemination, and reception are quite different processes. The reproductive justice focus of the pre-pregnancy care model did not erase reductionist thinking about women or about styles of health interventions. That is to say, while signaling an entreaty among experts to move beyond the silos that have reduced women to their reproductive status, the model continued to invoke and evoke entrenched ideas about women's ties to reproductive responsibility and about clinical solutions to social and medical problems. In drawing on the cultural and medical potency of thinking about women as potential mothers, the pre-pregnancy care framework amplified such thinking, even if it did so unintentionally. Those involved in producing the model might have hoped for a reproductive justice transformation, but their words also reveal how difficult it remains to disentangle ideas about (women's) social behavior and ideas about reproductive outcomes. This is because of the ways that our "cultural repertoire limits the available range of strategies of action"; culture can drive how "common sense" is defined.[6] We are willing to ask women and physicians to do quite a lot in the name of gendered clinical intervention; we are less willing to call on broad-based social changes that would give *all* people greater health security and put them at less risk at the outset. The evolution of pre-pregnancy care has partly played out the way it has because of the cultural resonance of thinking about women as mothers as well as our generalized hopes of assurance from preventive medical intervention.

On this point, pre-pregnancy care "made sense" to experts despite gaps in knowledge about its rationale and effectiveness, as detailed in Chapter 3. To the extent that defining women vis-à-vis their maternal status constituted not just a savvy *political* strategy but also an innovative *medical and public health* strategy that seemed to be a "natural path" forward reveals how cultural ideals about womanhood and motherhood are deeply linked. Conceptualizations of women as inherently reproductive animated not only policy strategy but also medical thinking about biological risk factors. Beliefs about reproductive risk were shrouded in cultural ideals about women and reproduction. In other words, conflating womanhood with motherhood was not just a guiding policy strategy, one that made for a compelling argument for reproductive justice, but a scientific logic as well—one that arranged reproductive-aged women's current behaviors in terms of their future maternal status. Pre-pregnancy care was politically expedient; it was also assumed to reduce risk.

RISK, POLITICS, AND THE PROBLEM OF ORDER

It is clear that thinking about reproductive risk is not one-dimensional. Policy initiatives can use reductionist and gendered frameworks while also attempting to advance reproductive justice. I have shown how the prevailing thinking about pre-pregnancy care has multiple layers and has been complicated by various concerns. While working to fasten ties between women's behaviors and reproductive outcomes, experts at times did mention men and did talk about the need for broader social change to improve maternal and child health. Yet, this nuance—revealed across Chapter 3 and Chapter 4—was flattened in the dissemination of the pre-pregnancy care messages analyzed in Chapter 5 and Chapter 6, as much of the roll-out was gendered and individualistic in nature. Clinical tools and health-promotion materials assigned burden to women and their behaviors rather than defining reproductive risk in a more expansive frame for reproductive justice. For all the progressiveness of vision among pre-pregnancy care experts, implementation of the initiative looked largely regressive to observers.

Thus, working without clear evidence to account for the pre-pregnancy care model but operating with political goals in mind, experts labored to define and deploy the pre-pregnancy care model. To recap, they formulated and fitted "facts" to the model, outfitting it with assumed "common sense" about women and reproduction. Tools were constructed, such as the "reproductive life plan," a device intended to assist clinicians and patients in assessing reproductive intentions and pre-pregnancy health risks. Advice books proliferated. That is, the new model produced knowledge at the same time that it produced medicine and markets. With a neoliberal tinge, pre-pregnancy health materials increasingly highlighted choice, empowerment, and individual responsibility for reducing reproductive risk, alongside racialized and gendered messages about reproductive responsibility. The pre-pregnancy care model became a new moral and scientific preoccupation with what women ingest, how they behave, and what their risks are *before* pregnancy.[7]

If experts were bound by how they perceived the problem of risk and how they perceived the politics of women's bodies, then their problems of knowledge were also problems of order.[8] If "risk-reducing interventions and risks themselves are often co-constructed and together constitute a coherent if largely invisible system of belief and practice,"[9] then medicine and public health worked together in this instance to produce a type of social control over women's bodies. As greater reproductive control became possible with widespread contraception in the mid-twentieth century, and as women's roles dramatically changed hence, the pre-pregnancy care model (as presented by health professionals) was positioned as a broad fix for pressing problems—medical, social, and political—including adverse birth outcomes, unintended pregnancies, and the politicization of women's health care. Policy prescriptions, clinical toolkits, and public-health campaigns defined and disseminated ways of thinking about reproductive responsibility, creating an ethic of anticipatory motherhood. This ethic exhorts women to act as if they are pregnant throughout their reproductive lives to reduce risks to future fetuses. The emergence of pre-pregnancy care is a case of knowledge construction and political maneuvering in which understandings about risk were bound by persistent cultural and medical tropes about women and maternal responsibility. To govern risk was to govern women. To promote anticipatory motherhood was to promote social order.

JUDGING THE SUCCESS OF THE PRE-PREGNANCY CARE MODEL

Widespread implementation of the CDC's recommendations for pre-pregnancy health and health care for the most part has not been accomplished.[10] Although women of reproductive age are beginning to receive more pre-pregnancy care than ever before,[11] not all women of childbearing age see themselves as needing such care.[12] Additionally, it is not entirely clear whether pre-pregnancy interventions have had a material impact on desired behavior changes.[13] Nevertheless, the model has effectively served as a bridging concept between the two worlds of reproductive care and maternity care.

Studies on pre-pregnancy care have skyrocketed over the past decade, as is shown in Chapter 1. These studies proliferated both in reproductive health journals and in maternal health journals, indicating that the concept of pre-pregnancy care interfaced with knowledge production in both spheres. The CDC's initiative—after initially facing backlash from feminist scholars—eventually enveloped experts who specialize in women's reproductive health. The second (2007) and third (2011) national summits on pre-conception health and health care convened top experts in the field, and deliberately included more women's health program leaders—seemingly organizing a united front for women's reproductive health and furthering the big-tent mission of pre-pregnancy care.[14]

Now pitched as a robust planning tool, the reproductive life plan concept, too, has traversed boundaries: organizations from Title X (representing the women's health "world" with a reproductive health focus) to midwifery and the March of Dimes[15] (representing the women's health "world" with a maternal and child health focus) have endorsed it. Reproductive life planning was highlighted as one of the Title X Family Planning Program Priorities in 2016, indicating that the reproductive care world had fully embraced the pre-pregnancy care model. The Title X Health and Human Services website stated that pre-pregnancy health services "are an important component of family planning services."[16] On the other end of the proverbial silo spectrum, the American College of Nurse-Midwives also posted a reproductive life plan on its website, indicating that "planning pregnancy leads to healthier pregnancies, healthier mothers, and healthier families."[17] The pre-pregnancy care model and its tools, namely the reproductive life plan, have morphed much more into addressing the problem of unintended pregnancies than attending only to birth outcomes. Although scholarly and popular critiques have berated pre-pregnancy care for its health-promotion messages, it is worth paying attention to the fact that women's health proponents have realized that the pre-pregnancy care strategy—even amid all its reductionist language—might be a useful schema not only for maternal and child health care but also for women's health care needs more broadly. Indeed, medical researchers are now thoughtfully working to situate reproductive life planning as a responsible intervention that does not infringe on women's reproductive autonomy.[18]

Few scholars have interrogated the overlap (or lack thereof) between maternal health care and reproductive health care. As I have argued in this book, this type of inquiry reveals much about how reproductive politics and semantics are shaped in America, affecting how we come to think and talk about women's bodies and behaviors. Studies about reproductive politics and health care agendas must more seriously consider the intricate relationship between maternal health and reproductive health—in both public policy and cultural discourse—to truly comprehend, promote, and value reproductive rights.[19] We must have nuanced conversations about points of overlap between maternal health and reproductive health, as this is the future—the point of future controversy and the point of future cooperation—in the realm of women's health. If we are going to improve population health, and treat women with respect while doing so, we need to be aware and beware of discourses that govern, rather than empower, women.

GOVERNING VERSUS EMPOWERING WOMEN

Governing women versus empowering women is a common trope in reproduction studies. Indeed, the zero trimester, as a socially constructed notion, reveals ongoing tensions in the reproductive arena—about how to advance reproductive justice without reducing women to baby vessels, about how to improve maternal and child health without sacrificing women's reproductive autonomy, and about how to expand women's reproductive opportunities without controlling their options and their bodies.

The rise of the pre-pregnancy care model in medicine and public health has surely been marked by paradox and contradiction. The idea was at once seemingly very new and apparently very old. It was at once completely perplexing (how many people contemplate the pre-pregnant body when thinking about pregnancy health?) and completely intuitive (of course it would "make sense" that good pre-pregnancy health would stimulate better outcomes). It was at once seemingly very bad for women's progress (treating women simply as reproductive vessels) and quite progressive (reconciling the often-bifurcated women's health arena). That there were multiple versions of conventional wisdom at work in the emergence of pre-pregnancy care—and that the public message didn't always match the intentions of pre-pregnancy care experts—reveals how difficult it is to craft reproductive agendas.

There always have been dualities and contradictions in reproductive health initiatives, with multiple narratives existing in tandem. Is expanding birth control a forward stride for female liberation or an insidious step toward population control?[20] Do long-acting contraceptives empower women to control their own fertility or do such technologies promote negative eugenics?[21] Do long-acting contraceptives coerce women to avoid reproduction or allow them access to health care they have long desired?[22] Do medical interventions over-medicalize and intrude in our lives; or do women want medical intervention in order to legitimize their pain and their problems?[23] These queries are representative of those that have plagued feminist reproduction scholars for some time. Pre-pregnancy care is no exception. In it, we see progress; we also see reversion. Expanded care for women might be good; defining women as pre-maternal might be less than ideal. Scholars and policy makers must be able to have discussions about the complexity of reproductive agendas and how to distribute information to the public, with an understanding that a thorny dialectic of innovation and digression might be how reproductive justice progresses in the long run. Dialogue is engendered (this book included) with every new reproductive initiative, allowing for the advancement of ideas and perceptions about how such agendas matter for women's lives.

EXPANDING RISK, EXPANDING BLAME

This nuanced endeavor is important in a culture that has given rise to a brutal ethos of mother-blaming, online and in public. People have a sense, be it accurate or not, of what "proper motherhood" is: whether to avoid alcohol while pregnant (or before pregnancy), whether to have a natural birth, whether to breastfeed (and for how long), how to parent—the list could go on and on. Medical and cultural messages can fuel dogmatic sentiments that do not make it easier for women to mother. Women, for the most part, are trying their best, with or without messages that make them feel guilty.

Maternal guilt is exacerbated by pervasive discourse in our society about maternal-fetal conflict. The current reproductive arena is one in which the rise of maternal-fetal medicine, fetal-surgery techniques, and technoscientific practices in the second half of the twentieth century shifted obstetrical gaze toward the fetus as an agent and patient separate from the mother.[24] Fetal risks in pregnancy began to be weighed against maternal risks.[25] In this vein, much contemporary ethical and cultural debate over reproduction has focused on abortion, prenatal technologies, or assisted-reproductive technologies, all of which bring to the fore conversations about potential maternal-fetal conflict.[26] The fetus is a salient object in our culture,[27] a fact that has smoothed the path for the cultural and medical emergence of the *future fetus*. Pre-pregnancy care has the potential to further expand social anxieties about maternal-fetal conflict, but such discourse now revolves around prospective procreation, as a woman's current behavior is seen as potentially negatively impacting a future fetus.

As Susan Markens and colleagues presented in a classic paper on reproductive practices and the maternal-fetal conflict, women's pregnancy *and* pre-pregnancy activities, such as dietary choices, are ever more affected by public dialogue about responsibility for fetal health.[28] Feminist scholars have argued that fetal rights and reproductive control discourse create an entrenched gendered social system, affecting even women who are not (or not yet) pregnant.[29] Cynthia Daniels posits that this type of discourse threatens women's autonomy and could perhaps "be invoked not just from the moment of fetal viability, or even from the moment of conception, but from the moment a woman becomes fertile."[30] Today, the "female body of childbearing age is redefined as the 'potentially pregnant' body."[31] As we continue to realize that we know little about the causes of birth outcomes, even amid major advances in reproductive science and technology, our paths of vision for progress must also attend to the potential for unintended consequences of the idea of the "potentially pregnant."

For instance, our cultural moment emphasizes perfect pregnancies and increasingly shames—even criminalizes—women for not achieving perfection. Under the auspices of "personhood" measures that categorize fertilized eggs, embryos, and fetuses as persons separate from the women carrying them, women today are on occasion prosecuted for experiencing stillbirths or miscarriages.[32] As mentioned in Chapter 6, if we take seriously that women's pre-pregnancy behaviors impact the health of a pregnancy, then it is not beyond the pale of imagination that women could be prosecuted for pre-pregnancy behaviors in future cases of adverse birth outcomes. There is a long history in the United States of blaming women for being "bad mothers" for all kinds of transgressions.[33] If women are defined as mothers before they are mothers, and even before they are pregnant, then all women of reproductive age are in a holding pattern for targeted examination.

Further, the mounting medical and social attempts to control conceptions and pregnancies might have prejudicial consequences for women who want to be pregnant. For individual women who experience an unwanted miscarriage, the rhetoric of pre-pregnancy care could exacerbate feelings of distress for early-pregnancy loss.[34] A woman erroneously might feel that she lost her pregnancy because of some behavior engaged in years, weeks, months, or days prior to conception. The reasons for miscarriage, like the causes of adverse birth outcomes, are not well understood by the medical community; most cases are likely of random distribution, calling into question any frame of blame or guilt. Also unaddressed in public discourse is the potential that the pre-pregnancy care framework could increase the abortion rate. A woman who is told that her pre-pregnancy behaviors or early pregnancy behaviors vastly increase her risk for an adverse birth outcome unfortunately might stop to consider whether to continue the pregnancy.

The pre-pregnancy care model must reckon, then, with its maternalist rhetoric—a rhetoric that can intensify guilt and blame even while it expands care. As much as pre-pregnancy advocates might insist that pre-pregnancy care is not limited to women who want to become mothers—after all, it is, in the literal sense, care before pregnancy regardless of whether an eventual pregnancy occurs—so much of the rhetoric around pre-pregnancy care is about improving birth outcomes, not about women's reproductive autonomy. In the way that prenatal care is care for women in expectation and anticipation of a birth, pre-pregnancy care is care for women in expectation and anticipation of an eventual pregnancy and, by extension, eventual motherhood.

ENVISIONING SOLUTIONS: THE SECOND NINE MONTHS

Many women will object to being treated as reproductive vessels. Many of the same women also might want access to comprehensive health care at each stage of their reproductive life. We should not only value women when they get pregnant, as the experts I interviewed so distinctly understood. We also should not continue the well-worn path of defining women as mothers to grant them access to care. Otherwise, any "year of the woman," to use the phrase summoned in Dr. Conry's speech at the opening of this chapter, might just be another year of the woman who is a potential mother. Maternalist visions for reproductive initiatives might actually conceal broader-based solutions to improve maternal and child health.

First, universal affordable health care is one such wide-ranging solution. To treat women across the life course would be to treat them as women, not as pre-mothers. To treat everyone is to treat women and men—indeed, all the potential reproducers in a society. That the experts implicitly knew that maternalism was the most expedient way to expand health access for women serves as an indictment on our society, as we have failed as a nation to make a basic social good—health care—available to everyone. Expanding health care options and access has defined the American style and vigor around pre-pregnancy care, in contrast with European countries. Although the United States has been the vanguard of pre-pregnancy care, the idea has not been limited to American physicians and policy makers. The first European meetings on pre-conception health and health care were held in Brussels in 2010. A notable distinction is that the focus in the United States has been largely on pre-conception *care* whereas much of the focus in Europe—where health care access is not such an impediment—has been on pre-conception *health* strategies.[35] The anxieties are different, reflective of our dissimilar investments into life course access to health care and health information.[36]

Second, other broad-based policies—such as universal paid family leave—would make a substantial difference in maternal and child health, contra to the ongoing ambiguity in evidence for a pre-pregnancy care framework. Such ambiguities in pre-pregnancy care are characterized by persistent uncertainty when dealing with the future. Although it might seem logical that healthy women have healthy babies, unhealthy women give birth to healthy babies all the time; healthy women can give birth to a baby with disabilities or health complications. Interventions that are risk-centered often do the work of "providing reassurance, reducing fear, and signaling responsibility for health," all the while trying to assert control over randomness.[37]

There is much we do not know about pregnancy, and this reality frustrates our sensibilities about controlling risk.[38] As sociologist Elizabeth Mitchell Armstrong writes about reproduction, "attitudes about risk are a way of coping with uncertainty, of dealing with the cruel randomness of nature and of life."[39] Pre-pregnancy care—as a new conceptual container for understanding reproductive risk and maternal responsibility—is a framework that has expanded social and medical control over reproductive risk through a focus on anticipation and taming the future. It is a deep human desire that aims to control and reduce risk to health—to our own health and to that of our children and future children. It also is a wide-ranging wish of society to ensure the well-being of future generations. In this spirit, the drive to tame risk is ubiquitous. In medicine and public health, the contemporary turn in such risk-reducing endeavors is to treat people as if they already have a disease, as if they are already risky—in the case of women of reproductive age, as if they are already pregnant. The temporal practice is not to wait for risk but to actively monitor any emergent factor that might introduce risk. Our trend toward anticipating risk and optimizing pregnancy is reflective of an obsession with looking ahead, with taming future uncertainties—in both medicine and in society.

Perhaps our obsession with looking ahead, however, blinds us to the present. What if policy attention were focused *more* on *maternal and child health*—that is, focusing on women once they are mothers and on babies after they are born? The United States is the only industrialized country that does not offer universal paid parental leave, which matters significantly for improving infant health.[40] Compared to other developed nations, public policy in the United States is hostile toward families, especially around issues of care.[41] Rich countries that have better maternal and child health outcomes than those in the United States have robust universal health care *and* allow ample time for families to focus on the health and well-being of their newborns and infants without fear of losing their jobs. In the United States we do neither.

An alternate focus to the zero trimester—an idea that is diffuse in its focus and almost unlimited in its scope—could be the "second nine months" as a temporal intervention. Early life matters, not only for babies, but also for mothers. Allowing women and families a "second nine months"—that is, paid leave for at least nine months after childbirth or adoption—would do much to humanize our maternal and child health system in the United States and bring us up to speed with other rich nations of the world that invest in parenthood and children. If and when parents return to paid employment, then providing workers with quality subsidized childcare would also be a step in this direction.

These policy recommendations might seem very "blue sky," but if we are truly to advance the well-being of our future generations, then we must discuss measures that would change the situation of women, children, and families in this country at a social-policy level, not only at an individualized one that has the potential to further exacerbate the blame and burden that women already feel in a society that does not—at higher institutional levels—seem to value the real needs of families and children.

If universal affordable health care and universal paid parental leave are not on the immediate policy horizon, and pre-pregnancy care continues to be an influential framework for—at the very least—improving health coverage for reproductive-aged women, then it is worth thinking earnestly about how to discuss reproductive risk and pre-pregnancy care in the most responsible manner possible. To conclude in this vein, I return to the case with which I began this book.

LOOKING AHEAD

In February 2016, reactions of confusion and mockery percolated into public discourse when the CDC issued its recommendation for all women of reproductive age to avoid drinking alcohol if they are not using contraception. *Slate* ran the headline: "CDC Says Women Shouldn't Drink Unless They're on Birth Control. Is it Drunk?!?" From *The Atlantic*: "Protect Your Womb From the Devil Drink. Let's talk about the CDC's bonkers new alcohol guidelines for women." It is probably safe to say that these recommendations were not successfully received in the public sphere. Why? First, the CDC's message was misleading about the temporality of risk. Pre-pregnancy drinking does not cause birth defects (nor does moderate drinking during pregnancy, for that matter).[42] This fact was quickly elicited by members of the media. Second, the message seemed clear-cut when, in fact, it is entirely unclear what causes many birth defects. Third, the message was gendered;

it mentioned only women and drinking, when studies are increasingly showing that alcohol-damaged sperm might lead to an increased risk of adverse reproductive outcomes. Finally, the CDC's alcohol recommendation is an excellent illustration of the contemporary public-health tactic of situating medical problems in individual behavior, and of the reinvigorated marriage between maternalism and medicalization. The CDC's message intimated that if women follow medical advice and change their lifestyles, then birth outcomes will improve. This line of thinking, however, does not get at root causes that are at the heart of public-health troubles. Policy interventions that provide citizens provide citizens with health care, paid parental leave, clean water, or unpolluted neighborhoods would have potentially huge impacts on the health of women, mothers, and children. Simply telling women of reproductive age not to have that glass of wine forestalls bigger discussions about what the causes of adverse birth outcomes really are—and what society should do about them.

Pre-pregnancy care might be an effective approach for some women and some men in some cases; but it is worth understanding and questioning how we label and define risk, and whether such labels and definitions disguise our abilities to see alternative approaches. So far, approaches to reducing reproductive risk have been gendered, uncertain, and narrowly focused. If women leading completely ascetic lives is the answer for the health of future generations, then we haven't looked far enough—we need to have a responsible conversation in public health and medicine about the interaction between behaviors and outcomes and how such notions currently are gendered, neoliberal, and individualistic, with often conflicting messages for women about how to go about their everyday lives.

Yet, there are different—and, I would argue, more conscientious—ways to approach issuing pre-pregnancy care recommendations about reproductive risk. To this end, I offer a contrasting contemporary case of reproductive risk. During the same month that it issued the alcohol warning, the CDC released its first report on the Zika outbreak,[43] a mosquito-borne virus associated with the risk of a birth defect: microcephaly in the infants of Zika-infected mothers. The CDC's report included special pre-pregnancy instructions for people of reproductive age. Compared to the alcohol message, these recommendations couldn't have looked more different. First, the report was clear about temporal risk. It indicated that, given the assessments at the time, women and men should wait to conceive if exposed to Zika, but the recommendations also indicated that there is no known risk to future pregnancies if Zika is contracted and resolved before a pregnancy. In other words, the report did not claim that having Zika today necessarily removes the chance of healthy reproduction in the future. Second, the report was fastidious in its explanation that much is unknown about the virus and its effects. The report highlighted uncertainty rather than masked it. Third, the message was aimed at men and women. In fact, the report indicated that it is important for exposed men to wait even longer than exposed women before conceiving—six months for men versus eight weeks for women—given that Zika seems to fester in semen. Finally, although not captured in this particular CDC report, public-health authorities have responded to Zika in part by working to eliminate the environmental risk agent (the mosquito), alongside warnings to women about travel and the risks of mosquito bites. In other words, the public health approach in this case has not been centered solely on telling women to change their behaviors. Whereas the alcohol warnings were disingenuous and paternalistic, the Zika recommendations could be interpreted as informative and empowering.

It is imperative that public-health messages include reliable information about health risks, including being clear about the temporal and causal direction of risks, acknowledging how much we really know (or don't know) about specific risks, accounting for the fact that risks are experienced by both men and women,[44] and understanding that profound risks are often beyond an individual's control. It is also crucial to document that some individuals—women and men—are at greater risk than others and to spend time working toward the difficult system-level solutions that might offer bigger rewards to maternal and child health than will deficient messages of behavior change. To govern reproductive risk is not necessarily to govern women. As seen in the Zika example, attention to risk can be framed in a diligent and cautious manner.

Although alcohol and infectious disease might be very different types of exposures, the public-health recommendations for each of these concerns have focused in part on alerting individuals to behavioral changes that might reduce risk to future pregnancies. The CDC's alcohol message—by proposing that a woman should think about a future baby when having a glass of wine today—seems utterly ridiculous. The Zika recommendations—

by navigating concerns about the relationship between exposures encountered in the pre-pregnancy period and potential risk of birth defects in future children—seem profoundly important. Such contrasting examples are instructive insofar as they highlight that there are different ways to navigate the growing pre-pregnancy care discourse that has permeated medical and public-health thinking about reproductive risk. Such avenues of action pivot on pressing questions: Do we continue on a neoliberal trend of individualizing risk and danger, simply telling women to get healthy in particular ways lest they harm a future pregnancy, even if this strategy doesn't get at the root of reproductive risk? Or, do we as a society take broad-based action to ensure the health and well-being of all people, including—hopefully—safeguarding the future generation in the process? We can acknowledge the prevailing uncertainty that characterizes life, and at the same time we can continue the vital work to improve maternal and child health outcomes in the United States.

We owe it to women to be forthright about reproductive risk and to let them experience life without thinking about their maternal status at every turn. We owe it to future children to think clearly about effecting real social change that will improve population health.

Notes

CHAPTER 1. SOMEDAY, NOW: PRECONCEIVING RISK
AND MATERNAL RESPONSIBILITY

1. Guttmacher Institute (2016).

2. Examples include Kate Storey, "The CDC Says You Shouldn't Drink If You're Not on Birth Control. Um, What?" *Cosmopolitan* (online), 2016 (Feb. 3), available at http://www.cosmopolitan.com/sex-love/news/a53108/young-women-alcohol -birth-control/ (accessed Feb. 25, 2016); Elizabeth Yuko, "The CDC Tells Women Not on Birth Control That They Can't Drink. Seriously?" *Ms. Magazine* Blog, 2016 (Feb. 5), available at http://msmagazine.com/blog/2016/02/05/the-cdc-tells -women-not-on-birth-control-that-they-cant-drink-seriously/ (accessed Feb. 25, 2016). Additional examples appear in Chapter 7.

3. Cited in Armstrong (2003, 201).

4. Roth (2000, 169–71).

5. Johnson et al. (2006).

6. Healthy Texas Babies campaign text, at https://www.dshs.state.tx.us /healthytexasbabies/Someday-Starts-Now.doc (accessed March 3, 2016).

7. Ibid.

8. A. Lynn, "Texas is Reminding Me I'm Just a Baby Vessel Again," *Nerdy Feminist* (blog), 2012 (Nov. 9), available at http://www.nerdyfeminist. com/2012_11_01_archive.html (accessed July 7, 2016).

9. The March of Dimes has a "12-Month Pregnancy Program for Educators," at http://www.marchofdimes.org/volunteers/12-month-pregnancy-program .aspx (accessed Nov. 23, 2016).

10. I use the term "women" in this book to stand in for those who have the capacity to become pregnant. I realize that this usage is to the exclusion of individuals who do not define themselves as women but who still have the capacity to get pregnant as well as individuals who define themselves as women but who cannot become pregnant. Regardless of actual capacity to get pregnant and no matter one's reproductive organs, the pre-pregnancy care model within medicine and public health purportedly speaks to any person who identifies as a woman. The term "woman" in this book captures the broad swath of the population that includes individuals who both identify themselves as women and have the reproductive organs commensurate with conceiving and gestating. "Women" and "men" also are the usual terms used in the health literature on this topic.

11. Claire Putnam, "Pregnant, Obese . . . and in Danger," *New York Times*, 2015 (March 28); Roni Rabin, "Patterns: Prenatal Vitamins May Ward Off Autism" *New York Times*, 2011 (June 13).

12. Crocker Stephenson, "Start Taking Care of Your Baby Before You Get Pregnant," *Milwaukee Journal Sentinel* online, 2011 (Nov. 14), available at http:// archive.jsonline.com/blogs/news/133824648.html (accessed April 10, 2017).

13. Miriam Stoppard, "Don't Focus on Getting Healthy While Pregnant—Do It Before Conceiving," *Mirror* (U.K.), 2016 (July 3), available at http://www.mirror .co.uk/lifestyle/health/dont-focus-getting-healthy-pregnant-8342693 (accessed July 6, 2016).

14. The only other reference I have found regarding an idea of a "zero trimester" is in a blog post about a couple's pre-pregnancy period in which the couple was actively trying to conceive. Available at: https://versionfourpointoh.word press.com/2007/12/06/the-whole-zero-trimester-thing/ (accessed June 8, 2016). In contrast to this reference, my usage of the term describes a more diffuse context for *all* reproductive-aged women, whether they are intending to get pregnant or not.

15. As an example of this messaging, the CDC's Third National Summit on Preconception Health and Health Care in 2011 in Tampa, Florida, started off by explaining to participants that pregnancy should be thought of as a yearlong endeavor (field notes). In honor of the summit, the Mayor of Tampa even declared June 13, 2011, to be "Preconception Health Day."

16. To be clear, some individuals involved in the CDC's pre-pregnancy work indicated to me that they are not in favor of the idea of promoting behavioral improvements only in the three months directly preceding a pregnancy, since such an approach is not long enough to combat a life course of behaviors (*see also* Moos 2003). Still, as referenced in this paragraph, organizations such as the March of Dimes promote the "twelve-month pregnancy" specifically. In this

book, I use the term "zero trimester" even more broadly than the twelve-month pregnancy idea, referring to the entire pre-reproductive zone of women's lives.

17. Gender theorist Kath Weston's idea of gender as a zero concept is instructive here. Weston writes "[Zero] does not pretend to make reference to something countable, something there, in any ontological sense. Zero marks absence and (perhaps) nothingness at the same time as it holds open a place for—represents the potential for—signification" (Weston 2002, 39). The idea of the zero trimester in pregnancy is hard to define, as it represents a "nothing" category (no pregnancy), but it is a place-holder, one that can be employed for social analysis. That is, zero's nonreferentiality opens up a critical perspective (Weston 2002, 49). Weston states that "a zero concept offers better possibilities for putting ever-changing social relations into perspective" (2002, 54).

18. See, e.g., Armstrong (2003); Daniels (1993); Taylor (2008).

19. Karp (2003).

20. Einhorn (2001).

21. Brink (2013).

22. The "fourth trimester" notion also focuses on supporting breastfeeding. See UNC Gillings School of Global Public Health's "Fourth Trimester Project," http://breastfeeding.sph.unc.edu/2015/12/15/the-4th-trimester-project/ (accessed Aug. 17, 2016).

23. I argue that looking at the margins of pregnancy (and, in this case, specifically prior to pregnancy) provides a clear vantage point on the social intersections of gendered reproduction. Most scholarly work on reproduction has examined pregnancy or fertility (including analyses of individuals' attempts to achieve pregnancy or, conversely, how the state attempts to dissuade pregnancies) or on women who are already mothers. By analyzing a discourse that targets women of reproductive age, I achieve further analytic leverage on the mechanisms of gendered inequality, as prior to pregnancy we might imagine a moment where both men and non-pregnant women are in the *same* pre-reproductive zone. See also Almeling and Waggoner (2013).

24. Johnson et al. (2006).

25. Using the MEDLINE (OCLC) database, which includes articles from medical and health journals from 1965 to present, I used multiple keyword searches to produce a graph of the number of articles on the topic of pre-pregnancy care published each year, 1980–2015. I limited the search to English-language results. These results include animal studies, although I focus on human studies for further analysis in this book. Results here are reported in raw numbers without regard to a denominator. The search was last updated May 2017. The following search terms were used: (kw: preconcept* and health) or (kw: pre-concept* and health) or (kw: preconcept* and care) or (kw: pre-concept* and care) or (kw: prepreg* and health) or (kw: pre-preg* and health) or (kw: prepreg* and care) or (kw: pre-preg* and care), with * denoting truncation. Thus, this search captured

all of the following terms used for "pre-pregnancy care" in the medical and health professional literature: preconception health/care; pre-conception health/care; preconceptional health/care; pre-conceptional health/care; preconceptual health/care; pre-conceptual health/care; prepregnancy (or prepregnant) health/care; pre-pregnancy (or pre-pregnant) health/care.

26. Johnson et al. (2006, 3).

27. Casper and Moore (2009, 67). Scholars have also cited pre-conception care and pre-conception messages as clear illustrations of biopolitical surveillance of the bodies of women of reproductive age (Gentile 2013; Mansfield 2012b).

28. Roni Rabin, "That Prenatal Visit May Be Months Too Late," *New York Times*, 2006 (Nov. 28).

29. January W. Payne, "Forever Pregnant," *Washington Post*, 2006 (May 16).

30. Amy Williams, "Warning: You Could Be Pre-Pregnant," *Ms. Magazine Blog*, 2011 (Jan. 26), available at http://msmagazine.com/blog/2011/01/26/warning-you-could-be-pre-pregnant/ (accessed April 10, 2017).

31. Wise (2008, S13).

32. Discussion of risk is often used politically to situate responsibility or blame (Douglas 1992).

33. This concept refers to the fear of letting others down, including, importantly for this discussion, *unknown* others. *See* Grant and Wrzesniewski (2010); Massi (2005). More broadly, for how emotion—including anticipation—shapes behavior, see Baumeister et al. (2007).

34. Chamberlain (1980).

35. Also cited in Cefalo and Moos (1995, 3).

36. Institute of Medicine (IOM) (1985, 15).

37. Department of Health and Human Services (DHHS) (1989, 26).

38. K. K. Barker (1998).

39. Ibid., 1068.

40. Armstrong (2000).

41. Atrash et al. (2006). Much of this increase was fueled by Medicaid expansions for pregnant women; the evidence was deemed weak as to whether such expansions improved birth outcomes (Howell 2001).

42. Atrash, Jack, and Johnson (2008). Recent data suggest that, despite recent declines in infant mortality, the United States is ranked twenty-sixth among 29 OECD countries in infant mortality (MacDorman et al. 2014). And maternal mortality is currently on the rise in the United States; the trend is in the opposite direction in other developed countries (MacDorman et al. 2016).

43. Armstrong (2000).

44. Ibid., 586.

45. Atrash et al. (2006).

46. Klerman (1990, 642, 634).

47. *See* Alexander and Kotelchuck (2001). For an excellent study on the clinical and cultural complexities surrounding preterm birth, see Bronstein (2016).

48. Finer and Henshaw (2006); Finer and Zolna (2011).

49. Coined by German biochemist Paul Ehrlich at the turn of the twentieth century, the term "magic bullet" refers to medicines that target and attack a specific disease while leaving healthy tissue unharmed. *See* Dubos (1959/1996); *see also* Davis (2016). Prenatal care has been loosely referred to as a medical care "magic bullet" in the sense that physicians have long believed that if they give women care during their pregnancy, all will be fixed. While the notion of "magic bullet" usually refers to *one* particular pharmaceutical intervention, prenatal care follows in the treatment paradigm of magic bullet fixes by holding to the idea that one particular clinical regimen will solve problems. That is to say, referring to prenatal care as a "magic bullet" does not reference a pharmaceutical treatment but rather a particular "treatment paradigm"—the idea that clinical care is the answer for all health and social problems. In this way, time and again, prenatal care has been pitched as a panacea—a one-stop universal remedy to cure all problems of reproductive risk during pregnancy.

50. Meckel (1990, 235).

51. The scholarly literature and health promotion materials often use the term "pre-conception"; I typically use the term "pre-pregnancy" to characterize the broader material shift toward thinking about the period prior to pregnancy as impacting birth outcomes. While the terms are not exactly synonymous (not every conception results in a pregnancy), they are often used synonymously in the literature and generally refer to the period prior to pregnancy. In my research on this topic over the years I have heard time and again, from both lay women and health professionals, that "pre-conception" is a confusing and not readily understood term. Some experts indicated in interviews that this term is cumbersome. I agree, and I prefer to use "pre-pregnancy" to facilitate communication and dialogue about the zero trimester. For an interesting discussion around this terminology, and its pros and its cons, see WHO (2012).

52. On infant mortality, see Lu and Johnson (2014). The CDC's push coincided with the first sustained period of lack of progress on infant mortality rates in the United States since the 1950s, which occurred during 2000–2005 (MacDorman and Mathews 2008, 2). On maternal mortality, see Lu et al. (2015). Public health scholars have long looked to primary health care for women as a means to reduce maternal morbidity and mortality rates (Rosenfield and Maine 1985).

53. Such as insurance coverage expansions that have promoted more prenatal-care visits. Prenatal care has also been bolstered by scientific advancements, such as ultrasound technologies that allow for intensive monitoring of fetal health, even if such enriched care does not offer further preventive benefits.

54. Armstrong (2000).

55. On the proclivity in contemporary medicine to focus on treatment over prevention and over holistic forms of healing the body, see Davis and González (2016).

56. *See, e.g.,* Armstrong (2003); Daniels (1993); Flavin (2009); Luker (1985); Paltrow (2013); Roth (2000).

57. *See, e.g.,* Keely (2012).

58. Friedman et al. (2016).

59. Opray et al. (2014).

60. A woman who continues a drug addiction into pregnancy is not necessarily going to end up giving birth to a baby with birth defects. For a rich analysis of the intersection of addiction, pregnancy, and other social and health risk factors, see Knight (2015). Knight notes that many women with opiate addictions do not realize that they are pregnant until advanced pregnancy symptoms appear. Also, concerns about drug use during pregnancy have not always resulted in predicted catastrophic outcomes, as has been found with the so-called (and debunked) crack-baby epidemic in the 1980s.

61. Johnson et al. (2006).

62. Although, researchers do note that smoking might delay or reduce fertility, and smoking occurring near the time of conception has been linked to cleft lip and cleft palate. *See* Department of Health and Human Services (DHHS) (2014).

63. This point is similar to Elizabeth Mitchell Armstrong's finding regarding fetal alcohol syndrome in which the problem of drinking became perceived as not just a problem for women at risk or for women drinking during pregnancy but rather the emphasis on not drinking was expanded to *all women* (Armstrong 2003, 200).

64. Atrash (2009); Lu et al. (2006).

65. The CDC's National Center on Birth Defects and Developmental Disabilities notes that the "causes of most major birth defects are unknown" (Centers for Disease Control and Prevention (CDC) 2008). Moreover, about 3% of babies born each year are defined as having structural birth defects; the CDC notes: "Although the evidence regarding known and suspected risk factors for birth defects continues to grow, the causes of the majority of birth defects remain unknown" (Centers for Disease Control and Prevention (CDC) 2015).

66. Wise (2008).

67. Xu et al. (2010).

68. Wise (2008, S15).

69. Chang et al. (2013). It is worth noting that it has been encouraging to pre-pregnancy care advocates that the infant mortality rate in the United States fell in 2005–2011, after the CDC and other organizations began targeting pre-pregnancy care. How much of this improvement in infant mortality was due to improved pre-pregnancy care is unknown. Part of this improvement is likely

driven by a reduction in the preterm birth rate—which includes many other variables unrelated to pre-pregnancy care, including unnecessary medical interventions around the time of birth, as mentioned here. *See* Abby Goodnough, "U.S. Infant Mortality Rate Fell Steadily from '05 to '11," *New York Times*, 2013 (April 17).

70. Robbins et al. (2014).

71. Ibid.

72. Ibid.

73. Xaverius and Salas (2013).

74. Mathews, MacDorman, and Thoma (2015).

75. Minino et al. (2007); MacDorman et al. (2016).

76. Solinger (2007).

77. Bish et al. (2012).

78. Anstey (2009).

79. The famous case is that of *Auto Workers v. Johnson Controls*, which dealt with the introduction of a "fetal protection policy." The Supreme Court ruled against Johnson Controls in 1991. *See* Daniels (1993, Chapter 3); Landsman (2009, 24).

Here, it is notable that pre-conceptional influences on fetuses have seeped into other arenas outside of medicine, namely that of law. Courts first recognized prenatal negligence to the fetus in 1946 (Robertson 1979), but the earliest preconception tort was in 1973 with the case *Jorgensen v. Meade Johnson Laboratories*. In this case, an infant plaintiff with Down syndrome claimed that her condition was due to contraceptives that her mother took prior to conceiving her (Babin 1979). In 1977, in *Renslow v. Mennonite Hospital*, an individual born prematurely and with brain damage claimed that her condition was the result of a blood transfusion (Rh-negative with Rh-positive) given to her mother prior to her conception (Robertson 1979). These two cases marked the beginning of a new phase of torts—prior to these cases, "recovery in every jurisdiction was limited to tortious conduct and injuries occurring after conception" (Steefel 1977, 621).

By 1990, the Arizona Supreme Court had defined three different types of "preconception torts" due to the great confusion surrounding preconception negligence (Silber 1992). Most preconception negligence cases involved individuals with birth defects claiming that the outcome was the result of some causal mechanism prior to conception. One of the well-known instances of the "preconception effect" was found in the ingestion of diethylstilbestrol (DES) among women. After its widespread release in 1941, DES was mostly used with the intent to prevent miscarriage; however, DES was also prescribed prior to 1941 to treat myriad reproductive conditions, including infertility (Bell 2009, 17). DES affected the adult health of daughters born to women who took it while trying to get pregnant. Some DES daughters have sued for negligence using a preconception torts framework (Monopoli 1995).

80. Rockhill, Kawachi, and Colditz (2000); Rose (1985).

81. Much social scientific attention has been paid to how life-course influences and exposures in early life matter for future outcomes (*see* Montez and Hayward 2011).

82. Waggoner and Uller (2015). It is yet unclear whether "epigenetics will fulfill its liberating potential or instead further racist or classist agendas" (Meloni 2016, 223).

83. Richardson et al. (2014).

84. Gentile (2013).

85. The 2006 *MMWR* document does not mention epigenetics research (Johnson et al. 2006).

86. Daniels (2006).

87. Antoniassi et al. (2016); Laubenthal et al. (2012).

88. Frey et al. (2008).

89. Roth (2000).

90. Almeling and Waggoner (2013).

91. Van der Zee et al. (2013).

92. Social scientific evidence points to social and environmental changes as mattering more to improving health than do changes in individual women's health behaviors. *See, e.g.,* Armstrong (2003); Currie and Walker (2011).

93. Luhmann (1993, Chapter 1).

94. *See, e.g.,* MacKendrick and Stevens (2016). Chapter 5 further discusses consumption and pre-pregnancy health.

95. Lupton (1995).

96. Goldstein (2001).

97. This principle has posed challenges for evidence-based public health interventions, especially those hinging on correlational evidence. *See* Weed (2004); Wolf (2011).

98. *See* Douglas and Wildavsky (1982); Giddens (1991). Risk and uncertainty often are treated synonymously as a way of thinking about potential harm (Lupton 1999/2006, p. 9).

99. Beck (1992); Castel (1991).

100. Armstrong (1995); Aronowitz (2009); Gillespie (2012); Greene (2007); Rosenberg (2009); Timmermans and Buchbinder (2010).

101. Rosenberg (2007).

102. Fosket (2010).

103. Rose (2007).

104. Clarke et al. (2003, 172).

105. Foucault (1978/1990, 140). *See also* Rabinow and Rose (2006). In the way that pre-pregnancy care is both the focus of public health policy and an ascendant medical framework for reducing risk, it could be termed what sociologist Steven Epstein calls a "biopolitical paradigm" (Epstein 2007, 17); Epstein defines

"biopolitical paradigms" as "frameworks of ideas, standards, formal procedures, and unarticulated understandings that specify how concerns about health, medicine, and the body are made the simultaneous focus of biomedicine and state policy."

106. Armstrong (2003); Kukla (2010); Mansfield (2012a).

107. Armstrong (1995, 402).

108. Adams, Murphy, and Clarke (2009, 248).

109. Ibid., 253.

110. With regard to epigenetics research, historian Sarah Richardson discusses the maternal body as an "epigenetic vector" (Richardson 2015). Furthermore, Martine Lappé notes in her research on autism science that the maternal body is increasingly the locus for social anxieties about autism and autism risk, both before and during pregnancy. She argues eloquently that such "spatial and temporal politics of risk and responsibility" may exacerbate surveillance of women's bodies (Lappé 2016).

111. Adams, Murphy, and Clarke (2009, 249).

112. Apple (2006); K. K. Barker (1998).

113. Lee (2007).

114. Duden (1993); Minkoff and Paltrow (2006); Petchesky (1987).

115. Armstrong (2003); Lupton (1999); Lyerly et al. (2009); Rapp (2000); Rothman (1993).

116. Armstrong (2007); Casper (1998).

117. Armstrong (2003); Markens, Browner, and Press (1997); Lupton (1999); Lyerly et al. (2009).

118. Zelizer (1985).

119. Hays (1996).

120. Wolf (2011, 71).

121. Badinter (2011); Blum (1999); Douglas and Michaels (2004).

122. Reich (2016).

123. Beck (1992); Giddens (1991); Wolf (2011).

124. MacKendrick (2014); Wolf (2011, especially Chapter 4).

125. Daniels (1997, 582–83).

126. Gentile (2013).

127. Lowe (2016).

128. Landsman (2009).

129. Boonstra et al. (2006).

130. Mathews and Hamilton (2002).

131. Available at http://www.census.gov/hhes/fertility/data/cps/historical.html (accessed Jan. 16, 2017).

132. Coale (1973).

133. See, e.g., Almeling (2011); Bell (2014); Franklin and Roberts (2006); Greil (1991); Markens (2007); Martin (2010).

134. Kukla (2005) historically documents how the uterus became public theater. The pre-pregnancy care framework changes the whole framework of visibility and risk, as women are monitored because they are *women*, not because they are pregnant women.

135. Eighty-five percent of women have at least one child in their lifetime. http://www.census.gov/hhes/fertility/data/cps/historical.html (accessed Jan. 16, 2017).

136. I followed the idea of "pre-conception care" or "pre-pregnancy care" through various spaces where knowledge about the idea was being produced and where cultural representations of the idea emerged. This approach lends itself to analyzing how medical knowledge, public health knowledge, scientific knowledge, health promotion, and cultural materials co-construct contemporary conceptualizations of pregnancy health and reproductive risk. As mentioned in the accompanying paragraph, I conducted in-depth interviews, ethnographic observation (sometimes participatory), historical research, as well as content analysis of medical and public-health literature, health-campaign materials, policy documents, and popular materials. For classic readings on the multisited ethnographic approach, see Marcus (1998); and Rapp (2000). More recent—and excellent—sociological examples of such an approach include Kempner (2014); and Shostak (2013).

137. The "core-set" model of field analysis has been used successfully when examining scientific or biomedical agendas that are forged by an identifiable group of experts (*see, e.g.,* Bliss 2012). In effect, I targeted the population of pre-pregnancy care experts in the nation for interviews, rather than sampling within a germane clinical or scientific specialty. As Catherine Bliss notes in her interview study with genomicists, referencing Latour, "core set analysis was specifically designed to get at black-boxed and unresolved knowledge," and it is an approach developed within interdisciplinary science studies (Bliss 2012, 8; *see also* Latour 1987). For a classic science-studies text that highlights the idea of the "core set" see Collins (1985), especially Chapter 6, "The Scientist in the Network: A Sociological Resolution of the Problem of Inductive Inference."

138. The CDC launched its Preconception Health and Health Care Initiative in 2004. In 2005, it convened the select expert panel to write the recommendations for pre-pregnancy care that were enumerated in the 2006 *MMWR*. In June 2006, the CDC reconvened most of the members of the expert panel and added more experts in substantive areas to hold the CDC's Proceedings of the Preconception Health and Health Care Clinical, Public Health, and Consumer Workgroup Meetings, which took place in Atlanta. Because this 2006 workgroup meeting included most of the select panel *in addition to* substantive experts in the field, I focused on this group for my in-depth interviews.

Focusing on the workgroups, rather than just the select panel also enabled me to capture more dissent and comparative dialogue. Because this workgroup was charged with taking the recommendations and implementing them through various arenas (clinical, public health, and consumer), this group was more diverse professionally and substantively than the select panel. Because this workgroup included most of the select panel, however, it also captures the words of those respondents who defined the pre-conception care recommendations before the initiative became more inclusive of various professional experts in the dissemination stage.

I contacted all of the individuals who were involved in the CDC's Preconception Care 2006 workgroups (n = 78). Interviews were conducted between February 2010 and June 2011. My full sample included 57 experts, including 43 women and 14 men. Represented in the sample were 52% (n = 12) of the CDC's clinical workgroup, 46% (n = 12) of the CDC's public health workgroup, and 48% (n = 13) of the CDC's consumer workgroup. Of these individuals, all but 7 overlapped with the CDC's select panel. After the Atlanta meeting, the CDC informally convened a policy workgroup, of which I interviewed all involved (n = 3). Moreover, one individual (n = 1) floated among the workgroups, and an additional group of individuals that I interviewed were not involved in the initial workgroups but were added to the leadership of the workgroups at a later date (n = 4). I did not detect a significant difference in expertise or professional discipline between those workgroup experts who responded to my interview requests and those who did not. Importantly, I interviewed all the workgroup leaders from the 2006 meeting except for one (workgroups had multiple designated leaders during this meeting); in total, I interviewed 10 of the 11 leaders, which matters significantly for the "core-set" field approach.

I also interviewed individuals who were not involved in the workgroups but who were involved in the initial select panel or the second select panel meeting convened by the CDC in 2007 (n = 11). The remaining individual that I interviewed (n = 1) was not involved in any of the panels or workgroups but held a high-level post with a women's health agency. This individual was indirectly involved in the CDC's pre-pregnancy initiative. I included this individual to gain some additional purchase on the questions of women's health backlash.

139. The final set of respondents included geneticists, obstetricians, public health specialists (some with an MPH degree, some with a DrPH degree), pediatricians, family practitioners, social scientists, epidemiologists, nurses, and policy experts. The respondents were not only clinicians, scientists, and researchers; many of them were also directors of high-profile organizations, government agencies, and academic medical departments. As such, in this book I am careful to retain anonymity by not always linking respondent quotes to an identifier such as occupation or gender. I also do not publish here a chart that lists academic specialty, race, or gender. The names of those who worked on the CDC's select panel and workgroups are publicly available, so I paid attention not to compromise internal confidentiality within my text (Tolich 2004). Additionally,

at times I refer to social scientists and other scientists only as "scientist" in the text. Because so few social scientists were represented, I found this prudent to protect confidentiality as well.

I interviewed ten key individuals in person, mostly in Boston, Washington, D.C., and at the CDC headquarters in Atlanta, Georgia. The remaining interviews were conducted and recorded over the phone; although, when performing participant observation at some meetings, I did meet some of these respondents in person. All respondents signed a consent form approved by the Brandeis University IRB. One respondent (Dr. Hani Atrash of the CDC) was too identifiable and too important to the study not to be identified. Thus, with Dr. Atrash's permission and with the permission of the Brandeis University IRB, Dr. Atrash signed a consent form that did not guarantee anonymity. This practice has been undertaken by other social scientists who study high-profile professional movements in the sciences (e.g., Bliss 2012; Reardon 2004).

In-depth interviews are important because they distinguish the "contingent," or informal discourse of the scientists from the more formal space of scientific publications (Gilbert and Mulkay 1984) and allow for triangulation of various kinds of information. Some aspects of scientific advancement are not always part of the formal knowledge production repertoire (Latour and Woolgar 1979; Star 1983). The objective of the in-depth interviews was to elicit detailed responses in various categories to ascertain the respondent's views on pre-conception (or pre-pregnancy) care. These data then were used in qualitative analysis.

The analytic coding strategy used in analyzing interview data followed the principles of grounded theory method (Charmaz 2006; Glaser and Strauss 1967). Grounded theory uses an inductive technique of coding, which is appropriate for a study on the emergence and consequences of a new medical and health strategy. This technique also involves constant data comparison to document and unearth the social context and processes around the phenomenon of interest. Constant comparison is an analytic approach that uses explicit coding in conjunction with theory development (Glaser 1965, 437). My analytic strategy also was influenced by a new extension of the grounded theory method, that of the social words framework (Clarke 2005; Clarke and Star 2007), which "focuses on meaning-making amongst a group of actors—collectivities of various sorts—and on collective action" (Clarke and Star 2007, 113).

All of my interviews were transcribed. The qualitative-analysis software program, ATLAS.ti, was used to facilitate data analysis. Both transcriptions and memos were closely read for the purpose of developing codes for emergent themes. When a code emerged in several instances and across interviews, I retraced to make sure that the codes were maintaining meaning and consistency across contexts.

140. One limitation of my approach is the generalizability of the study's findings to the broader profession of health experts who work on maternal and child health

issues. To the extent that I focused on a clearly defined cross section of a specific group of crucial actors who can speak to their role throughout this shift, and simultaneously examined the literature of this professional arena (Hilgartner and Bosk 1988), however, I am able to speak to the *process and meaning* by which a particular health strategy emerges among the professional elite whose work seeps into the public and medical discourse. An obvious drawback to this method of studying the elite is the lack of non-dominant voices, but because this project is interested in the project of this elite (or, at least, successful) group, this is not a drawback to the method for this particular project (*see* Bucher 1962/1972; Zetka 2008b).

Additionally, in focusing attention to how knowledge has shifted within maternal and child health toward pre-pregnancy risk factors, the design of my analysis privileges the words of experts insofar as it is their words, their publications, and the dissemination of their ideas on which I rely. An obvious critique is that this approach ignores women themselves—how they are embracing or resisting such ideas. This is an important point, and another book could and should be written on women's narratives and perspectives on pregnancy health risk in the twenty-first century. My analysis in this book first seeks to fill major gaps in our understanding about the origins of this care framework, and may offer important insights into how women are beginning to navigate this new reproductive-risk terrain.

141. Jasanoff (2004); Shapin and Schaffer (1985).

CHAPTER 2. FROM THE WOMB TO THE WOMAN: THE
SHIFTING LOCUS OF REPRODUCTIVE RISK

1. Chamberlain (1980, 29). *See also* Atrash, Jack, and Johnson (2008); Freda, Moos, and Curtis (2006); Jack et al. (2008).

2. Smith-Rosenberg and Rosenberg (1976/1997).

3. Quoted in Cefalo and Moos (1995, 1).

4. In addition to using the MEDLINE database with search terms provided in Chapter 1, I focused on four prestigious medical journals for historical context: *British Medical Journal* (from 1840), *Lancet* (from 1823), *The New England Journal of Medicine* (from 1812), and *Journal of the American Medical Association* (from 1883). Much of the early history discussed here was found in searchable electronic databases, especially that of *The New England Journal of Medicine*, formerly known as *The New England Journal of Medicine and Surgery* and *The Boston Medical and Surgical Journal*. In these nineteenth-century and early twentieth-century journals, I searched for any article that was related to prenatal care or that included phrases such as "before conception" and "before pregnancy," because "pre-pregnancy (or pre-conception) care" was not yet a term used in the literature. I follow Hilgartner and Bosk (1988) in using medical and

scientific journal publications as representative of a public arena in the formation of formal medical knowledge. Additionally, I read through old obstetric
texts as well as historical monographs that detail aspects of the history of prenatal care or maternal and child health in the United States. Such references
appear throughout this chapter.

5. Armstrong (2003, 15).

6. "Dropsy of the Amnion and Foetus" (1824, 360).

7. Bennet (1829).

8. Oakley (1984, 23).

9. Smith-Rosenberg and Rosenberg (1976/1997).

10. Ibid., 27–28.

11. Ibid., 25.

12. Ibid., 27 (emphasis added).

13. Armstrong (2003, 29).

14. Dewees (1825, xi) (emphasis added).

15. Clarke (1873).

16. Zschoche (1989).

17. Roberts (1997).

18. Smith-Rosenberg and Rosenberg (1976/1997, 55).

19. Ibid., 68.

20. Worcester (1900, 362).

21. "Case Showing the Importance of Early Manual Examination in Cases of
Threatened Abortion" (1824, 121).

22. Ibid., 124.

23. Channing (1825, 155).

24. Ibid., 156.

25. Stebbins (1887, 445) (emphasis in original).

26. "Reports of Societies" (1889).

27. "Reports of Societies" (1894, 594).

28. Cumston (1895, 283).

29. Post (1889).

30. "An Epitome of Current Medical Literature" (1912, 58).

31. Speert (1980).

32. Brandt (1985, 11).

33. Ibid., 19.

34. In 1899, Michigan became the first state to enact such a law. By 1913,
seven states had similar laws on the books. Only men were required to undergo
these examinations, lest a woman' character be affronted (Brandt 1985, 19–20).

35. Brandt (1985, 19).

36. Ibid., 140.

37. Ibid., 147.

38. Ibid., 147–48.

39. Ibid., 147.

40. Ibid., 149–50.

41. Ibid., 150.

42. Oakley (1984, 11).

43. Ibid., 25.

44. Helme (1907, 421) (emphasis added).

45. Ibid., 425.

46. Ballantyne (1901, 813).

47. Oakley (1984, 46).

48. Ibid., 64.

49. Ibid., 64.

50. Ibid., 84.

51. Ibid., 86.

52. Skocpol (1992, 2) (emphasis added).

53. K. K. Barker (1998).

54. This specific history is revisited in Chapter 6.

55. Oakley (1984, 87).

56. Ibid., 87.

57. From the *Lancet*, quoted in Oakley (1984, 86).

58. Ballantyne (1905).

59. BMJ (1904, emphasis added). Ballantyne also dedicated some of his writing to the understanding of syphilis and primary prevention. As he wrote in his 1902 volume, *Manual of Antenatal Pathology and Hygiene: The Foetus*, "there is a large mass of evidence to show that syphilis, and possibly other morbid conditions, may arise in the foetus through paternal influence or through maternal influence *prior to conception*" (Ballantyne 1902, 288, emphasis added).

60. Zabriskie (1929), quoted in Thompson, Walsh, and Merkatz (1990).

61. BMJ (1934, 221).

62. "Reports of Societies" (1903, 379).

63. Taussig (1937, 110).

64. Adair (1941, 647) (emphasis added).

65. Goethals (1940, 64) (emphasis added).

66. Adair (1936).

67. Adair (1940).

68. Ibid., 7.

69. Duster (2003, 32).

70. Stern (2005).

71. JAMA (1932).

72. Ibid., 1906.

73. Toombs (1923).

74. Ibid., 35.

75. *See, e.g.*, Takeshita, Peng, and Liu (1964).

76. March of Dimes (2002).

77. The following citations are illustrative, not exhaustive: Atrash, Jack, and Johnson (2008); Johnson and Gee (2015).

78. Hewitt (1939, 417).

79. JAMA (1940, 638).

80. Gold (2001).

81. Coale (1973).

82. JAMA (1966, 38).

83. Friesen (1970, 495).

84. Broadly, obstetrics was in a period of disciplinary upheaval entering the post-WWII years due to general surgeons' claims that obstetrics was not living up to its surgical skill set, putting ob-gyn legitimacy at risk (Zetka 2008b). Of course, when professions encounter fissures regarding their legitimacy, jurisdictional claims are forged over particular problem arenas (Abbott 1988).

85. Shwartz (1962).

86. Gold (1955); JAMA (1952); Van Ness (1955).

87. Van Ness (1955, 3255).

88. Gold (1955, 247).

89. Cross (1961).

90. Russell (1962, 83).

91. Sociologist James R. Zetka detailed how the specialty of obstetrics-gynecology began a concerted effort in the 1970s to become the "women's physician," situating itself as women's primary care physicians to restructure the specialty to have more access to women's problems upstream and thus to control their own referrals (Zetka 2008a).

92. Russell (1962, 1025).

93. JAMA (1966).

94. Ibid., 38.

95. Friesen (1970).

96. Ibid., 495 (emphasis added).

97. Arney (1982, 51).

98. Friesen (1970, 497).

99. For an excellent historical overview of early folic acid studies and the intersection between the rise of pre-pregnancy care and folic acid, see Al-Gailani (2014).

100. Smithells, Sheppard, and Schorah (1976). Folic acid is one of the B-vitamins; its naturally occurring form, folate, is found in foods such as leafy green vegetables. Neural tube defects refer to a class of birth defects wherein the development of the spinal cord or the brain in the fetus is devastatingly or fatally affected, such as in the condition of spina bifida.

101. Al-Gailani (2014, 282).

102. Smithells et al. (1980), also detailed in Al-Gailani (2014).

103. Al-Gailani (2014, 282).

104. Smail (1981) quoted in Al-Gailani (2014, 280).

105. Mills et al. (1989).

106. Wald et al. (1991).

107. Centers for Disease Control and Prevention (CDC) (1992).

108. Quoted in Al-Gailani (2014, 284).

109. Al-Gailani (2014).

110. Ibid., 285.

111. Ibid., 279.

112. Wald (1993, 126–27).

113. Junod (2003).

114. Honein et al. (2001).

115. Junod (2003, 56).

116. Oakley (1984, 166).

117. Earlier in the 1960s, enthusiasm increased for studying and viewing human embryology, or the very early stages of development after fertilization and implantation. The cover of *Life* magazine in 1965, on which the photographer Lennart Nilsson published color pictures of the embryonic and fetal stages of development in humans, became a cultural icon. In writing about this cover, Elizabeth M. Armstrong argued that "this kind of visualization had the effect of socializing pregnancy, of making the experience commonly accessible to all rather than a private, interior experience of the pregnant woman alone" (Armstrong 2003, 195). Of course, medical and social attention to the embryo is not new. As Kristin Luker revealed in her history of the first "right-to-life" movement in the late nineteenth century, physicians worried that women "did not know that the embryo was alive because they subscribed to the 'outmoded' doctrine of quickening" (Luker 1985, 21–22).

118. Human embryology studies have existed since the nineteenth century, most notably under the direction of Dr. Wilhelm His in Germany. Ballantyne, in his *Manual of Antenatal Pathology and Hygiene: The Foetus*, wrote that at around the fortieth day of gestation, the "new organism takes on a form which can be recognized as distinctly human" (Ballantyne 1902, 80). Not until systematic collections of specimens in the 1940s and 1950s, and with the publication of systematic syntheses of "appropriate data" in the 1970s, did knowledge significantly move forward about the *timing* of human embryological development (O'Rahilly 1979). Indeed, prior to the 1970s, "embryological resumes [were] vague [and] often quite unreliable in regard to timing" (O'Rahilly and Gardner 1971).

119. Muller and O'Rahilly (1985).

120. *See, e.g.,* Barker (1995).

121. Oaks (2001); Reagan (2010).

122. D. J. P. Barker (1998); *see also* Almond and Currie (2011); Petronis (2010).

123. Chamberlain (1980, 29).

124. Lumley et al. (1980).

125. Williams (1980).

126. BMJ (1981).

127. Ibid., 685.

128. Baker (1981); Barrison et al. (1981).

129. Barrison et al. (1981, 1332).

130. Speller (1981, 859).

131. Cartier et al. (1982); Seller (1982).

132. Steel et al. (1982, 355).

133. Heslin and Natow (1984, 469).

134. Krasner (1984, 181–82).

135. Hollingsworth, Jones, and Resnik (1984).

136. *Lancet* (1985).

137. Ingamells (1987).

138. Jewell (1990, 351).

139. Page (1981, 858).

140. It is worth noting here that physicians also might not have been invested in the first few weeks post-fertilization, before knowing whether the pregnancy has "taken," given the very high rates of spontaneous abortion (miscarriage). Almost one in five pregnancies end in miscarriage; some estimates are as high as 50% of pregnancies. Miscarriage represents the majority of pregnancy loss in America, and most miscarriages occur in the first trimester (Layne 2003, 11). It is a relatively common occurrence among women of reproductive age. *See also* Lara Freidenfelds, "Misunderstanding Miscarriage," Blog, 2014, available at https://larafreidenfelds.com/2014/03/28/misunderstanding-miscarriage/ (accessed July 13, 2016); and the March of Dimes on miscarriage, http://www .marchofdimes.org/complications/miscarriage.aspx (accessed July 13, 2016).

141. Page (1981).

142. Reader and Grudzinskas (1985).

143. Klerman and Reynolds (1994).

144. Jack (1995).

145. Moos and Cefalo (1987, 63).

146. Rosenblatt (1989).

147. Atrash et al. (2008).

148. Klerman (1990).

149. Alexander and Kotelchuck (2001, 308); *see also* Lu et al. (2003).

150. Strong (2000).

151. Skocpol (1992).

152. K. K. Barker (1998).

153. Moos (2006).

154. Strong (2000).

155. Institute of Medicine (IOM) (1985, 15).

156. Department of Health and Human Services (DHHS) (1989).

157. BMJ (1991, 1174).

158. Scholars of reproduction have noted the historical consistency of societies defining the special place of women as the "nation's mothers." Illustrative references, although not exhaustive, include Armstrong (2003); and Yuval-Davis (1997).

159. Cefalo and Moos (1988).

160. Cefalo and Moos (1995).

161. Jack and Culpepper (1990).

162. National Center for Health Statistics (NCHS) (2001).

163. Ibid.

164. The ACOG statement argued that any multi-specialty effort to provide pre-pregnancy care should be "directed by the obstetrician-gynecologist" (American College of Obstetricians and Gynecologists (ACOG) 1995, 201). As this chapter demonstrates, however, attention to pre-pregnancy care was not clustered within obstetrics alone.

165. Hellerstedt et al. (1998).

166. Moos et al. (1996).

167. Herman and Perry (1992/1997).

168. March of Dimes (2002).

169. Lu and Halfon (2003); Misra, Guyer, and Allston (2003).

170. At https://www.cdc.gov/mmwr/about.html (accessed July 14, 2016).

171. Rosenbaum (2008).

172. Johnson et al. (2006, 4).

173. Ibid., 2.

174. Ibid., 2.

175. Ibid., 19.

176. Contemporary pre-pregnancy care literature is also concerned with inter-pregnancy care, although its visibility is not as bright as that of pre-pregnancy care. Representative articles on inter-conception care include Johnson and Gee (2015); and Lu et al. (2006).

CHAPTER 3. ANTICIPATING RISKY BODIES: MAKING SENSE OF FUTURE REPRODUCTIVE RISK

1. Armstrong (2003); Aronowitz (2015); Lupton (1995); Rosenberg (2007).

2. For just a few excellent examples in this vein, *see* Armstrong (2003); Aronowitz (1998); Barker (2005); Epstein (2007); Kempner (2014); and Wailoo (2011).

3. *See also* Armstrong (2003); Wolf (2011).

4. Jack and Culpepper (1990, 1149); the authors cited diabetes and maternal PKU as conditions amenable to preconception intervention.

5. Freda and Patterson (1994, 19).

6. See methods overview and notes in Chapter 1 for a discussion about the "core set" approach. Respondents were active in one or more of the CDC's expert workgroups from the Select Panel on Preconception Care. This core set of experts was instrumental in forging a new clinical and social definition of reproductive risk. Following the Select Panel's definition, the concept and terminology gained greater recognition and legitimacy, with increased visibility for pre-pregnancy care in science and society.

7. See methods note in Chapter 1 for more information about interview recruitment strategy and details.

8. Cefalo and Moos (1988).

9. Moos and Cefalo (1987).

10. Moos is still active in the initiative and the National Summits on preconception health and health care. Cefalo passed away in 2008.

11. Atrash later moved to work with the Maternal and Child Health Bureau.

12. Johnson et al. (2006, 10).

13. See Chapter 1 for discussion of "magic bullets" in medicine.

14. Hays (1996); Wolf (2011).

15. Several experts mentioned that it is impossible to conduct a randomized trial to test enhanced medicalization of pregnancy; however, such studies have been attempted. In one example, public health scholar Lorraine V. Klerman and her colleagues set up an experimental design at the University of Alabama Birmingham in the late 1990s to test the effectiveness of additional prenatal interventions among low-income African American women. Their study found no difference in incidence of low birth weight between the control group and the group that received enhanced prenatal care access and services (Klerman et al. 2001), calling into question how much good medicalization can do. One puzzle, then, at the heart of the rise of the pre-pregnancy care framework is that if clinical interventions during pregnancy had not worked, according to the experts, why would clinical intervention prior to pregnancy do any good?

16. Ballantyne (1902), also quoted in Oakley (1984, 47).

17. Quoted in Oakley (1984, 50).

18. Hilgartner (2000); Star (1985).

19. Cunningham et al. (2014).

20. *See, e.g.,* Franklin and Roberts (2006); Landsman (2009); Lappé (2014); Lupton (1999); Stern (2005).

21. Until fairly recently, the fetus as a "perfect parasite" was a typical metaphor used in medical discussions about pregnancy, nutrition, and fetal development. For a popular overview, see Paul (2010).

22. Creager (2013, Chapter 8).

23. Moreover, and as already mentioned, physicians historically have dissuaded women from presenting for care during their first trimester because so

many early pregnancies do not "take" (i.e., many early pregnancies result in miscarriage, sometimes even before a woman ever realizes she was pregnant). It is a cultural practice, too, for women to wait beyond the embryonic phase of gestation to announce the pregnancy, for much the same reasons. It is potentially devastating for women and men to have to explain to friends and loved ones that the pregnancy vanished. Lynn Morgan writes of the cultural ascendance of the embryo in her book (Morgan 2009); these cultural and medical shifts also have exacerbated experiences of pregnancy loss (Layne 2003).

24. The focus on "awareness" also emerged in the medical literature; a 1993 March of Dimes publication titled "Toward Improving the Outcome of Pregnancy: The 90s and Beyond," for example, included a chapter on "reproductive awareness" as a "basic health promotion strategy" (March of Dimes 1993, 12).

25. *See, e.g.,* Aiken et al. (2016); Higgins, Hirsch, and Trussell (2008); Luker et al. (1999); Trussell, Vaughan, and Stanford (1999).

26. Stevens (2015).

27. Mann (2013). *See also* Geronimus (2003).

28. Fennell (2011).

29. For example, the United States has been found to have greater rates of unintended pregnancy and teenage pregnancy than those of Canada and Europe (Darroch et al. 2001).

30. Also, focus was on women's lack of reproductive awareness prior to pregnancy to avoid unwanted pregnancies, but attention rarely was paid to a woman's desires should she conceive an unwanted pregnancy. The experts tended to discuss pregnancy as if it were a done deal. That is, a major assumption in the pre-pregnancy care model is that women should prepare their bodies for pregnancy, so that the pregnancy will be healthy, no matter what a woman's intentions might be regarding an actual pregnancy. In theory, if the pre-pregnancy care approach succeeded at the population level, then fewer abortions would be necessary. If women planned their pregnancies and engaged in pre-pregnancy care, the framework presumes, pregnancies would be desired and healthy. This, of course, ignores the many complicated and nuanced reasons that women need abortion and reproductive care.

31. Armstrong (2003).

32. Klerman (1997).

33. Atrash et al. (2006, S4).

34. I am drawing on the rich literature in medicalization theory; for a book that provides an excellent overview, see Conrad (2007).

35. Pharmaceuticalization is a key component of contemporary discussions of medicalization. *See* Bell and Figert (2015).

36. Zola (1972).

37. *See* Aronowitz (2015).

38. Greene (2007).

39. Conrad (2007). Anticipatory health practices have the potential for expanding medicalization of latent or previously invisible "risk factors" (*see* Brown 1995; Shostak 2010).

40. For example, "normal sadness" becomes clinically-treated depression (Horwitz and Wakefield 2012), shyness becomes a disorder (Lane 2007), or hyperactive children become considered a medical problem (Conrad 2007).

41. Clarke et al. (2003).

42. Adams, Murphy, Clarke (2009).

43. *See also* Conrad and Waggoner (2017).

44. Aronowitz (2009).

45. Scholars have pointed to how anticipation in child health-risk discourse centers on maternal responsibility, especially in pregnant women (*see, e.g.,* Lappé 2014; Lappé 2016). My work highlights the anticipation of risk in a future body; that is, risk discourse here is not focused on a pregnant body and a fetal body, but rather on a potentially pregnant body and a not-yet-existent fetus.

46. Kempner (2014, 20). *See also* Markens (1996); Martin (1987/2001).

47. Epstein (2007).

48. Swidler (1986).

CHAPTER 4. WHITHER WOMEN'S HEALTH? REPRODUCTIVE POLITICS AND THE LEGACY OF MATERNALISM

1. It is worth noting that in the CDC's *MMWR* document, Recommendation 7 and Recommendation 8 discussed relevant policy (specifically, Medicaid) and programs (notably Title V and Title X) discussed in this chapter (Johnson et al. 2006).

2. The grass-roots women's health movement was also most active during the 1970s and early 1980s, calling attention to the patriarchal medical establishment's historically dismissive treatment of women. Women themselves were calling for greater control over their reproductive lives and bodies, and it was questionable whether they would trust the medical establishment to assist in this endeavor. *See* Ruzek and Becker (1999).

3. For example, the Division of Reproductive Health, within the National Center for Chronic Disease Prevention and Health Promotion, is separate from the division that focuses on birth defects, within the National Center on Birth Defects and Developmental Disabilities.

4. Becker (1963, 148–50).

5. Beckett (1996).

6. Aronson (1984).

7. Best (1987).

8. Armstrong (1998); Armstrong and Abel (2000); Rosenberg (1976/1997).

9. Epstein (2007).

10. AbouZahr (2003).

11. Faludi (1991).

12. Rosenfield and Maine (1985).

13. Klerman (1990, 634).

14. Wilcox (2002).

15. AbouZahr (2003, 18).

16. Klerman (2006).

17. For an eloquent argument on this point, see Misra and Grason (2006).

18. Gordon (1994); Skocpol (1992).

19. Skocpol (1992, 2) (emphasis added).

20. Solinger (2007).

21. Much of this history has been documented, but I want to briefly focus on how the maternal health "camp" came to be known as a separate entity from general "women's health." For good historical overviews, see Gordon (1994); Hutchins (1994); Koven and Michel (1993); Lesser (1985); Skocpol (1992).

22. Skocpol (1992, 10).

23. K. K. Barker (1998; 2003).

24. Information for much of this history comes from the work of Hutchins (1994); Lesser (1985); and Skocpol (1992).

25. See Meckel (1990); Skocpol (1992, 509).

26. Skocpol (1992, 505-506).

27. Skocpol (1992).

28. Rothman (1978); also discussed in Skocpol (1992, 515).

29. See Hutchins (1994); van Dyck (2010).

30. Of note, Title V defined mothers and children as dependents. The way in which "needs" get defined is influential for the ways in which citizens perceive certain populations, as "entitled" or "drains" on the state, for instance (Fraser 1989).

31. The Children's Bureau was disabled over time. See Hutchins (1994, 698).

32. Lesser (1985).

33. Quadagno (2015, 79).

34. Rosenbaum (2008); see also Salganicoff and An (2008). Jill Quadagno has pointed out that Medicaid modernization (expanding Medicaid eligibility to include additional groups) has been a trend since the 1980s (Quadagno 2015).

35. Quadagno (2015, 82); Quadagno further notes in this chapter, citing the work of health policy expert Colleen Grogan, that starting in 2014, Obama's Affordable Care Act expanded "Medicaid's mandatory coverage groups by

requiring that participating states cover nearly all people under age 65 with household incomes at or below 138 percent of the FPL."

36. An exemplary history is found in Gordon (2007). *See also* Jacqueline E. Darroch (2006). Such references highlight not only the history of family planning in America but also the emergent and ongoing controversies presented by advances in family planning methods and women's changing roles over the course of the last century.

37. Gold (2001).

38. Information for this discussion is drawn mostly from Gold (2001); and Darroch (2006).

39. Gold (2001).

40. See Joffe (2009) for a great discussion of abortion and reproductive care in America and the stigma that accompanies it.

41. On the rise of fetal rights and fetal visibility, see Daniels (1993); Dubow (2011); Duden (1993).

42. Again, there is some overlap between the silos in practice; for example, abortion procedures take place in maternal health care settings that are outside of family planning clinics. Still, the depiction of the reproductive silos as persistently separate realms is part of the narrative of why pre-pregnancy health and health care is needed.

43. Brandt and Gardner (2000).

44. Clarke (1998).

45. Social scientists have a critical interest in the concept of "boundaries." The idea of "boundary-work" (Gieryn 1983) describes the ways in which scientists forge delineations between themselves and non-scientists to establish credibility and authority (Gieryn 1999). Lamont and Molnár (2002) note that much of the boundary-work scholarship focuses on the differences that boundaries highlight. Susan Leigh Star's work, conversely, emphasizes the importance of "boundary objects" that actually facilitate and bridge differences. This formulation is what informs my discussion of pre-pregnancy care as a bridging concept. Bowker and Star (1999) write that classification systems and tools function to coordinate knowledge and action. *See also* Star and Griesemer (1989). Moreover, pre-pregnancy care is a kind of collective effort that took place in face of resistance from other experts and social critics (*see* Frickel and Gross 2005).

46. Swidler (1986).

47. Koven and Michel (1993, 2) (emphasis in original).

48. The role of health experts and providers sometimes might be more nuanced than the surface suggests (*see also* Markens 2013).

49. "Non-Hispanic white women average about 2.7 lifetime pregnancies per woman, compared with 4.2 pregnancies per woman for non-Hispanic black and Hispanic women" (Ventura et al. 2008, 5).

50. It is worth noting that the folic acid findings in the late twentieth century—that folic acid taken around the time of conception could prevent birth defects—was hailed at the time as "exciting" because of how it might be able to reduce the need for abortions during a time of upheaval for reproductive politics (Al-Gailani 2014, 282).

51. As Epstein (2007, Chapter 3) notes about tacit coalitions, individuals approach the big umbrella with different foci and variable opinions.

52. Epstein (2007).

53. Gurr (2015).

54. Luna and Luker (2013); *see also* Ross (2006); Solinger (2007).

55. Verbiest et al. (2016).

56. Bridges (2011).

57. Joffe and Reich (2015, 240).

58. Solinger and Nakachi (2016, 27).

59. This concept draws on Wolf (2011).

60. Weisman (1998, 195).

61. Armstrong (2003); Yuval-Davis (1997).

62. Brush (1996).

63. Weisman (1998, 198).

64. For an excellent discussion of this conundrum, see Daniels (1993), especially 90–95.

CHAPTER 5. GET A REPRODUCTIVE LIFE PLAN!
PRODUCING THE ZERO TRIMESTER

1. Emphasis added to the title word "before."

2. Murkoff and Mazel (2009, viii).

3. Available at http://www.prnewswire.com/news-releases/ept-introduces-revolutionary-preconception-health-test-to-help-reduce-risk-of-preterm-labor-258284921.html (accessed May 7, 2014). On the establishment of the home pregnancy test as a common diagnostic tool, see Robinson (2016).

4. Franklin and Roberts (2006); Markens (2013); Roberts (2009).

5. Cullum (2003, 543).

6. Ibid. (emphasis added).

7. Ibid., 548.

8. Jack (1995). Of course, these days most women take a pregnancy test at home, meaning that there are perhaps fewer clinical moments that are explicitly reproductive in nature in which physicians can "do" pre-pregnancy care.

9. Atrash, Jack, and Johnson (2008, 584).

10. Cullum (2003).

11. Krissy Brady, "7 Nutrients Your Body Needs if You Think You Might Get Pregnant Soon," *Women's Health* Magazine, 2015 (July 30), available at http://www.womenshealthmag.com/mom/prenatal-vitamins (accessed Nov. 13, 2015); Editors, "Healthy Pregnancy Timetable," *Shape* Magazine, 2009 (April 23), available at http://www.shape.com/lifestyle/mind-and-body/healthy-pregnancy-timetable (accessed Nov. 13, 2015); Laurel Leicht, "Thinking of Getting Pregnant? You Might Want to Stop Taking This Type of Medicine, *Glamour* Magazine, 2015 (July 20), available at http://www.glamour.com/health-fitness/blogs/vitamin-g/2015/07/pregnant-birth-defects-antidepressants (accessed Nov. 13, 2015).

12. At www.everywomancalifornia.org (accessed Jan. 16, 2017).

13. At www.everywomanfl.com (accessed Jan. 16, 2017). Florida has been included as part of Every Woman Southeast, available at http://everywomansoutheast.org/partners/florida (accessed May 10, 2017).

14. At http://everywomannc.com (accessed Jan. 16, 2017).

15. http://www.onekeyquestion.org/ (accessed Jan. 16, 2017).

16. http://beforeandbeyond.org/toolkit/ (accessed Jan. 16, 2017).

17. Ibid. (emphasis in original).

18. For an excellent article that shows how providers aim to subvert gendered and individualized notions of responsibility for reproductive risk, see Stevens (2016).

19. MacDorman and Mathews (2008).

20. Finer and Zolna (2011).

21. Malnory and Johnson (2011).

22. For instance, the initiative organized a special journal issue on preconception health policy in *Women's Health Issues* (2008, 18(6), supplement).

23. Link and Phelan (1995).

24. Roberts (1997); *see also* Armstrong (2003).

25. Moos et al. (1996).

26. Moos (2006, 157); *see also* Moos et al. (2008).

27. Moos et al. (2008, S281).

28. Field notes from webinar, 2010.

29. At http://everywomannc.org/your-health/rlp/are-you-ready/ (accessed May 3, 2017).

30. At http://www.cdc.gov/preconception/reproductiveplan.html (accessed Dec. 9, 2016).

31. At http://www.marchofdimes.org/professionals/12-month-pregnancy-program.aspx (accessed Dec. 9, 2016).

32. Mittal, Dandekar, and Hessler (2014).

33. Mayo Clinic, "Preconception Planning," http://www.mayoclinic.org/healthy-lifestyle/getting-pregnant/in-depth/preconception/art-20046664 (accessed Dec. 9, 2016).

34. Nelson et al. (2016).

35. Lois Bloebaum, "Utah Preconception Campaign," Utah Department of Health, 2010, available at http://www.poweryourlife.org/wp-content /uploads/2010/08/Lois-Bloebaum-BSN-MPA-ppt.pdf (accessed May 4, 2017).

36. Chuang et al. (2015).

37. Charlotte Hilton Andersen, "Study Shows Half of Women Don't Know Basic Facts About Baby-Making," *Shape* Magazine, 2014 (Jan. 27), available at http://www.shape.com/lifestyle/mind-and-body/study-shows-half-women-dont -know-basic-facts-about-baby-making (accessed Nov. 13, 2015).

38. Deborah Gaines, "A Preconception Checklist," *Parents* Magazine, 2010 (Nov.), available at http://www.parents.com/getting-pregnant/pre -pregnancy-health/general/preconception-health-checklist/ (accessed Dec. 9, 2016).

39. Leslie Pepper, "Your Pre-Conception Diet Makeover," *Parents* Magazine [n.d.], available at http://www.parents.com/getting-pregnant/pre-pregnancy -health/diet/pregnancy-nutrition-diet-health-plan/ (accessed Nov. 13, 2015).

40. Leah Fessler, "4 Foods You Should Avoid Now if You Want to Get Pregnant Later," *Women's Health* Magazine, 2014 (Aug. 18), available at http://www .womenshealthmag.com/mom/pre-pregnancy-foods-to-avoid (accessed Nov. 13, 2015).

41. Marisa Cohen, "Want a Baby Someday? How to Preserve Your Fertility," *Women's Health* Magazine, 2009 (Aug. 16), available at http://www.womens healthmag.com/health/women-fertility (accessed Nov. 13, 2015).

42. Hallie Levine, "The Pregnancy Health Crisis No One's Talking About," *Redbook* Magazine, available at http://www.redbookmag.com/life/mom-kids /advice/a16836/pregnant-and-obese/ (accessed Nov. 13, 2015).

43. For an excellent piece on how breastfeeding—as another reproductive endeavor that aims to optimize childhood health outcomes—became a middle-class, privileged "project" for women, see Avishai (2007). Vaccine refusal also fits this mold among some privileged women, evoking a contemporary neoliberal ethos vis-à-vis childhood health risk (Reich 2014).

44. Murkoff and Mazel (2009, 2).

45. Sussman and Levitt (1989).

46. Herman and Perry (1992/1997).

47. Fournier and Fournier (1980).

48. Ibid., xi.

49. Ogle and Mazzullo (2011).

50. Lu (2009).

51. Much research focuses on how stress impacts pregnancy outcomes. It is worth noting, however, that pre-conception biomarkers related to chronic stress have not been found to be related to adverse birth outcomes (Wallace et al. 2013).

52. Lu (2009, 218).

53. Ibid., 221.

54. From the March of Dimes catalog, at http://www.marchofdimes.com/catalog/product.aspx?productid=4977&categoryid=170&productcode=37-2170-07 (accessed Oct. 28, 2010).

55. Wise (2008).

56. Foucault (1988).

57. Lupton (1999, 67).

58. Beck (1992).

59. Giddens (1991, 117).

60. *See* Adams, Murphy, and Clarke (2009); Rose (2007).

61. Choiriyyah et al. (2015).

62. Daniels (1997, 582).

63. Almeling and Waggoner (2013).

64. Armstrong (2003).

65. Campo-Engelstein et al. (2016).

66. Frey et al. (2008).

67. Lu (2009, 259).

68. Markham Heid, "5 Reasons She's Not Getting Pregnant," *Men's Health* Magazine, 2014 (Sept. 16), available at http://www.menshealth.com/health/why-she-cant-get-pregnant (accessed Nov. 13, 2015).

69. Wolf (2011, 76).

70. At http://www2.cdc.gov/ncbddd/faorder/images/099-6230_a.jpg (accessed Jan. 26, 2010).

71. Editors of *Shape.com*, "Essential Facts about Fertility and Infertility," [n.d.], available at http://www.shape.com/lifestyle/mind-and-body/fertility-infertility (accessed Nov. 13, 2015).

72. Latham Thomas, "How to Prepare for Pregnancy Now (Even Though You're Nowhere Close to Actually Being Pregnant!)" *Essence* Magazine, 2015 (April 17), available at http://www.essence.com/2015/04/17/prepare-future-pregnancies (accessed Nov. 13, 2015).

73. Duggan (2003); Harvey (2007).

74. Bay-Cheng (2015).

75. Lupton (1995); Petersen and Lupton (1996).

76. *See*, for instance, Epstein (2007).

77. Jasanoff (2004).

78. Metzl and Kirkland (2010).

79. MacKendrick (2014); Szasz (2007).

80. An analysis of online pre-conception health messages in 2015 also found that pre-conception recommendations are highly gendered and individualized (Thompson et al. 2017).

81. Clarke (2004, 71). *See also* Han (2013); MacKendrick (2014); Pugh (2009); Rothman (1989).

CHAPTER 6. PROMOTING MATERNAL VISIONS:
GENDER, RACE, AND FUTURE BABY LOVE

1. This quotation and similar ones below are taken from the Centers for Disease Control and Prevention's "Show Your Love" campaign. This text was posted online in 2013 but is now no longer active.

2. Moos (2010).

3. The campaign division between intenders and non-intenders is discussed in Lynch et al. (2014).

4. Centers for Disease Control and Prevention (CDC), "Preconception Care and Health Care," Atlanta, GA, 2013, available at https://www.cdc.gov /preconception/showyourlove/ (accessed April 2013).

5. I conducted this analysis in April 2013.

6. Charmaz (2006).

7. *See, e.g.,* Mamo, Nelson, and Clark (2010).

8. Kabat (2008).

9. Hoppe (2013).

10. Conrad (1994).

11. Lupton (1995).

12. Brandt and Gardner (2000); *see also* Krieger (1994); Pearce (1996).

13. Nettleton (1996, 34).

14. Ibid., 34, 36.

15. Brandt and Rozin (1997, 1).

16. Brandt and Gardner (2000).

17. *See, e.g.,* Campbell (1999); Daniels (1997); Kukla (2010); Lupton (2012); and Oaks (2001).

18. Armstrong (2003); Balsamo (1999); Daniels (1993); Markens, Browner, and Press (1997); Paltrow (2013); Waggoner (2013).

19. Available at http://www.cdc.gov/preconception/video/planner/index.html (accessed April 6, 2017).

20. *See* Beck and Beck-Gernsheim (1995); Foucault (1988).

21. Foucault (1988, 18).

22. Beck (1992). *See also* Giddens (1991); Lupton (1999).

23. Giddens (1991, 47).

24. *See* Layne (2003).

25. Adams, Murphy, and Clarke (2009); Clarke et al. (2010); Rose (2007).

26. MacKendrick (2014).

27. Gentile (2013); Kukla (2010); MacKendrick (2014); Mansfield (2012a).

28. "Show Your LOVE! Steps to a Healthier Me and Baby to Be!" Document #CS23 8162-B. Centers for Disease Control and Prevention, Atlanta.

29. "Show Your LOVE! Steps to a Healthier Me!" Document #CS23 8988-A. Centers for Disease Control and Prevention, Atlanta.

30. Ibid.

31. Pre-conception health materials, by highlighting the importance of planning future maternity, aim to facilitate all pregnancies as wanted pregnancies and thereby also aim, to some degree, to avoid entirely the politics of abortion. *See* Waggoner (2013).

32. Giddens (1991).

33. This practice extends the growing trend of "gifting" pregnant women things from their future baby; see Han (2013, 167) on the growing trend of how pregnant women at baby showers are now given gifts "from" their babies.

34. Cancian (1986).

35. Almeling (2011); Hird (2007); Ragoné (1999).

36. Berend (2012, 914).

37. Available at https://www.cdc.gov/preconception/showyourlove/documents/radioscript-30second-nonplanner-solo-speaker.pdf (accessed May 3, 2017).

38. Almeling and Waggoner (2013).

39. All three videos were posted at http://www.cdc.gov/preconception/showyourlove/videos.html (accessed April 6, 2017).

40. Of course, not all relationships are racially homogeneous—so it should not be assumed that Jada's partner would necessarily be black—but, in contrast to the representation of the white woman with her partner, the lack of symmetry with Jada's situation is worth noting.

41. Collins (2005).

42. *See, e.g.,* Markens (2012).

43. *See, e.g.,* Solinger (1992/2000).

44. Colen (1995, 78).

45. Ginsburg and Rapp (1995, 3).

46. Collins (2005).

47. Roberts (1997).

48. Ladd-Taylor and Umansky (1998); Markens (2007).

49. Finer and Zolna (2011); MacDorman and Mathews (2008).

50. *See* McLanahan and Percheski (2008).

51. Gálvez (2011).

52. Jones et al. (2013); Williams and Sternthal (2010).

53. Blum (1999).

54. Kukla (2005).

55. Lewis (1997, 61).

56. Apple (2006, 22).

57. Lee (2007); Litt (2000).

58. Hays (1996, 8).

59. Wolf (2011, 18).

60. Lowe (2016, 2).

61. Paltrow and Flavin (2013, 333).

62. Flavin (2009).

63. Badinter (2011).

CHAPTER 7. GOVERNING RISK, GOVERNING WOMEN: ANTICIPATORY MOTHERHOOD AND SOCIAL ORDER

1. Conry (2013).

2. Pre-pregnancy researchers are increasingly calling for greater gender equity in the pre-pregnancy realm (*see, e.g.,* Casey et al. 2016).

3. There no doubt are individuals who deftly travel across these boundaries. One of my own mentors, Dr. Lorraine V. Klerman, was renowned in the maternal and child health community. She received prestigious lifetime achievement awards from several maternal and child health organizations and has publishing prolifically on family planning services. Others, such as Dr. Milton Kotelchuck—of the eponymous index for prenatal care provision—did the same. But despite the *ability* to wade into the waters on both topics, it takes initiative and courage to do so given the state of reproductive politics in the United States.

4. Epstein (2007).

5. Mathews and Hamilton (2002).

6. Swidler (1986, 284).

7. Armstrong (2003); Kukla (2005).

8. Bliss (2012); Jasanoff (2004); Shapin and Schaffer (1985).

9. Aronowitz (2015, 6).

10. Johnson et al. (2015).

11. Bello, Rao, and Stulberg (2015) found that in ambulatory care settings, women of reproductive age have been receiving more pre-conception care than prior to 2005, when the CDC began promoting pre-conception care. This finding, though, largely was attributed to provision of prescription contraception.

12. One Dutch study found that, even among those trying to conceive, women often do not see themselves as a target group for pre-pregnancy care (Van der Zee et al. 2013). Moreover, health experts and officials have tried to improve pre-pregnancy care messaging to appeal to more women (as evidenced by a 2013 special issue of *American Journal of Health Promotion* 27(sp3)).

13. In a study about the relationship between pre-pregnancy messages and pre-pregnancy behaviors, authors found that folic acid counseling resulted in pre-pregnancy vitamin use but that messages about other behavioral changes such as dieting, drinking, and smoking were not associated with changes in behavior (Oza-Frank et al. 2015). Furthermore, the Cochrane Database of Systematic Reviews has found that pre-pregnancy health promotion is largely ineffective (Whitworth and Dowswell 2009).

14. I am drawing on Epstein's (2007) term.

15. Available at http://www.marchofdimes.org/pregnancy/planning-your
-pregnancy.aspx (accessed April 7, 2017).

16. Available at http://www.hhs.gov/opa/title-x-family-planning/initiatives
-and-resources/preconception-reproductive-life-plan/ (accessed April 7, 2017).

17. Available at http://www.midwife.org/ACNM/files/ccLibraryFiles
/Filename/000000001514/ Developing%20a%20Reproductive%20Life%20
Plan.pdf (accessed April 7, 2017).

18. Callegari et al. (2016).

19. For a fabulous argument about how reproductive rights must be inclusive—to not only focus on family planning and abortion but also to increase focus
on the rights of pregnant women who want their babies—see Paltrow (2013,
17–21).

20. This question has been asked specifically of Margaret Sanger's work in the
early days of Planned Parenthood.

21. Roberts (1997).

22. For example, Mann (2013) has shown how young women want medical
intervention because it affords better attention, care, and other benefits.

23. Barker (2005); Kempner (2014).

24. Armstrong (2007); Casper (1998).

25. Armstrong (2003); Lupton (1999); Lyerly et al. (2009).

26. *See, e.g.,* Luker (1985); Rapp (2000); Rothman (1993); Wertz (2001).

27. Duden (1993); Minkoff and Paltrow (2006).

28. Markens, Browner, and Press (1997).

29. Paltrow (2013).

30. Daniels (1993, 4).

31. Balsamo (1999, 239).

32. Paltrow (2013).

33. Ladd-Taylor and Umansky (1998).

34. *See* Lara Freidenfelds (2014), "If the IUD Is an Abortifacient, Then So Is
Chemotherapy and Lunch Meat." Blog. Available at https://nursingclio
.org/2014/05/21/if-the-iud-is-an-abortifacient-then-so-is-chemotherapy-and-lunch
-meat/ (accessed April 7, 2017).

35. A report from the Preconception Health and Health Care Initiative news-
letter from the 1st European Congress on Preconception Care and Preconception
Health held in Brussels in 2010 included the following statement, "Most striking
from a US perspective is the degree to which our efforts are focused on access,
while virtually all European systems have provided coverage and a medical home
for each woman and man. In addition, discussions focused on a preconception
visit versus a preconception health strategy."

Furthermore, some European programs appear to be more about infertility,
later childbearing, and epigenetics, whereas in the United States the focus
consistently has been on expanding health care access and reducing unintended

pregnancy rates. That said, notable recent examples such as a pre-conception report out of Scotland do indicate that programs and reports are increasingly highlighting the optimization of care and the importance of planning among reproductive-aged individuals (Sher 2016). Also, see the PrePreg Network in Europe, available at http://www.pubcare.uu.se/forskning/vardvetenskap /prepreg_network/ (accessed April 7, 2017).

36. "Preconception care" is also emerging in the global health literature as a way to provide babies with better chances for survival and well-being, as well as a strategy for reducing maternal mortality (WHO 2012; WHO et al. 2012). Definitions of "preconception care" in these WHO reports mirror that of the CDC's 2006 report, showing the broad influence of the CDC's work to promote the concept.

37. Aronowitz (2015, 5–6).

38. *See* Armstrong (2003, Chapter 7).

39. Armstrong (2003, 217).

40. Nandi et al. (2016); *see also* Burtle and Bezruchka (2016).

41. Williams (2012).

42. Armstrong (2003).

43. Available at http://www.cdc.gov/mmwr/volumes/65/wr/mm6512e2 .htm?s_cid=mm6512e2_w.htm (accessed Dec. 9, 2016).

44. It is worth noting that de-gendering the zero trimester might just exacerbate guilt and blame for *both* men and women if such change is not met with broader social changes that address what puts people at risk in the first place.

Bibliography

Abbott, Andrew. 1988. *The System of Professions: An Essay on the Division of Expert Labor*. Chicago: The University of Chicago Press.

AbouZahr, Carla. 2003. "Safe Motherhood: A Brief History of the Global Movement 1947–2002." *British Medical Bulletin* 67(1): 13–25.

Adair, Fred L. 1936. "Undergraduate Obstetric Education." *Journal of the American Medical Association* 106: 1441–42.

———. 1940. "Preconceptional Care." *The American Journal of Surgery* 48: 7–13.

———. 1941. "The Management of Pre-Eclampsia." *New England Journal of Medicine* 224: 644–49.

Adams, Vincanne, Michelle Murphy, and Adele E. Clarke. 2009. "Anticipation: Technoscience, Life, Affect, Temporality." *Subjectivity* 28(1): 246–65.

Aiken, Abigail, R. A., Sonya Borrero, Lisa S. Callegari, and Christine Dehlendorf. 2016. "Rethinking the Pregnancy Planning Paradigm: Unintended Conceptions or Unrepresentative Concepts?" *Perspectives on Sexual and Reproductive Health* 48(3): 147–51.

Alexander, Greg R. and Milton Kotelchuck. 2001. "Assessing the Role and Effectiveness of Prenatal Care: History, Challenges, and Directions for Future Research." *Public Health Reports* 116(4): 306–16.

Al-Gailani, Salim. 2014. "Making Birth Defects 'Preventable': Pre-Conceptional Vitamin Supplements and the Politics of Risk Reduction." *Studies in History and Philosophy of Biological and Biomedical Sciences* 47: 278–89.

Almeling, Rene. 2011. *Sex Cells: The Medical Market for Eggs and Sperm.* Berkeley: University of California Press.

Almeling, Rene and Miranda R. Waggoner. 2013. "More and Less Than Equal: How Men Factor in the Reproductive Equation." *Gender & Society* 27(6): 821–42.

Almond, Douglas and Janet Currie. 2011. "Killing Me Softly: The Fetal Origins Hypothesis." *Journal of Economic Perspectives* 25(3): 153–72.

American College of Obstetricians and Gynecologists (ACOG). 1995. "ACOG Technical Bulletin—Preconceptional Care." *International Journal of Gynecology & Obstetrics* 50(2): 201–07.

"An Epitome of Current Medical Literature." 1912. *British Medical Journal* 2(2704): 57–60.

Anstey, Erica Hesch. 2009. "Contaminating the Hallowed Maternal Body: A Feminist Approach to the Dilemma of Endocrine Disruptors on Maternal and Child Health." *Journal of the Association for Research on Mothering* 11(1): 167–79.

Antoniassi, Mariana Pereira, Paula Intasqui, Mariana Camargo, Daniel Suslik Zylbersztejn, Valdemir Melechco Carvalho, Karina H. M. Cardozo, and Ricardo Pimenta Bertolla. 2016. "Analysis of the Functional Aspects and Seminal Plasma Proteomic Profile of Sperm from Smokers." *BJU International* 118(5): 814–22.

Apple, Rima. 2006. *Perfect Motherhood: Science and Childrearing in America.* New Brunswick: Rutgers University Press.

Armstrong, David. 1995. "The Rise of Surveillance Medicine." *Sociology of Health & Illness* 17(3): 393–404.

Armstrong, Elizabeth M. 1998. "Diagnosing Moral Disorder: The Discovery and Evolution of Fetal Alcohol Syndrome." *Social Science & Medicine* 47(12): 2025–42.

———. 2000. "Lessons in Control: Prenatal Education in the Hospital." *Social Problems* 47(4): 583–605.

———. 2003. *Conceiving Risk, Bearing Responsibility: Fetal Alcohol Syndrome and the Diagnosis of Moral Disorder.* Baltimore: The Johns Hopkins University Press.

———. 2007. "What Happened to the M in MFM? The History and Evolution of Maternal-Fetal Medicine." Paper presented at the American Sociological Association Annual Meeting, New York, New York.

Armstrong, Elizabeth M. and Ernest L. Abel. 2000. "Fetal Alcohol Syndrome: The Origins of a Moral Panic." *Alcohol & Alcoholism* 35(3): 276–82.

Arney, William Ray. 1982. *Power and the Profession of Obstetrics.* Chicago: The University of Chicago Press.

Aronowitz, Robert A. 1998. *Making Sense of Illness: Science, Society, and Disease.* Cambridge: Cambridge University Press.

————. 2009. "The Converged Experience of Risk and Disease." *The Milbank Quarterly* 87: 417–42.

————. 2015. *Risky Medicine: Our Quest to Cure Fear and Uncertainty.* Chicago: The University of Chicago Press.

Aronson, Naomi. 1984. "Science as Claimsmaking: Implications for Social Problems Research." In *Studies in the Sociology of Social Problems,* edited by J. Schneider and J. Kitsuse. Norwood, NJ: Ablex. Pp. 1–30.

Atrash, Hani. 2009. "Preconception and Interconception Health: The Why, the What, and the How To." Paper presented at the Before, Between, and Beyond Pregnancy: Understanding Preconception and Interconception Health Conference, Fort Worth, Texas. February 27.

Atrash, Hani, Brian W. Jack, and Kay Johnson. 2008. "Preconception Care: A 2008 Update." *Current Opinion in Obstetrics & Gynecology* 20(6): 581–89.

Atrash, Hani, Brian W. Jack, Kay Johnson, Dean V. Coonrod, Merry-K. Moos, Phillip G. Stubblefield, Robert Cefalo, Karla Damus, and Uma M. Reddy. 2008. "Where Is the 'W'oman in MCH?" *American Journal of Obstetrics & Gynecology* 199(6): S259–S65.

Atrash, Hani K., Kay Johnson, Myron Adams, Jose F. Cordero, and Jennifer Howse. 2006. "Preconception Care for Improving Perinatal Outcomes: The Time to Act." *Maternal and Child Health Journal* 10: 3–11.

Avishai, Orit. 2007. "Managing the Lactating Body: The Breast-Feeding Project and Privileged Motherhood." *Qualitative Sociology* 30: 135–52.

Babin, Peter B. 1979. "Preconception Negligence: Reconciling an Emerging Tort." *Georgetown Law Review* 67: 1239–62.

Badinter, Elisabeth. 2011. *The Conflict: How Modern Motherhood Undermines the Status of Women.* Translated by A. Hunter. New York: Metropolitan.

Baker, C. C. 1981. "Preconception Clinics (Correspondence)." *British Medical Journal* 283: 1055.

Ballantyne, J. W. 1901. "A Plea for a Pro-Maternity Hospital." *British Medical Journal* 1(2101): 813–14.

————. 1902. *Manual of Antenatal Pathology and Hygiene: The Foetus.* Digitized by the Internet Archive in 2010 with funding from Open Knowledge Commons and Harvard Medical School. New York: William Wood & Company.

————. 1905. *Manual of Antenatal Pathology and Hygiene: The Embryo.* New York: William Wood & Company.

Balsamo, Anne. 1999. "Public Pregnancies and Cultural Narratives of Surveillance." In *Revisioning Women, Health, and Healing: Feminist, Cultural, and Technoscience Perspectives,* edited by A. E. Clarke and V. L. Olesen. New York: Routledge. Pp. 231–53.

Barker, D. J. P. 1995. "Fetal Origins of Coronary Heart Disease." *British Medical Journal* 311(6998): 171–74.

———. 1998. "*In Utero* Programming of Chronic Disease." *Clinical Science* 95: 115–28.

Barker, Kristin. K. 1998. "A Ship upon a Stormy Sea: The Medicalization of Pregnancy." *Social Science & Medicine* 47(8): 1067–76.

———. 2003. "Birthing and Bureaucratic Women: Needs Talk and the Definitional Legacy of the Sheppard-Towner Act." *Feminist Studies* 29(2): 333–55.

———. 2005. *The Fibromyalgia Story: Medical Authority and Women's Worlds of Pain.* Philadelphia: Temple University Press.

Barrison, I.G., I.M. Murray-Lyon, J. Waterson, J. Wright, and I. Lewis. 1981. "Preconception Clinics (Correspondence)." *British Medical Journal* 283: 1332.

Baumeister, Roy F., Kathleen D. Vohs, C. Nathan DeWall, and Liqing Zhang. 2007. "How Emotion Shapes Behavior: Feedback, Anticipation, and Reflection, Rather Than Direct Causation." *Personality and Social Psychology Review* 11(2): 167–203.

Bay-Cheng, Laina Y. 2015. "The Agency Line: A Neoliberal Metric for Appraising Young Women's Sexuality." *Sex Roles* 73(7): 279–91.

Beck, Ulrich. 1992. *Risk Society: Towards a New Modernity.* Los Angeles: SAGE.

Beck, Ulrich and Elisabeth Beck-Gernsheim. 1995. *The Normal Chaos of Love.* Translated by Mark Ritter and Jane Wiebel. Cambridge: Polity.

Becker, Howard S. 1963. *Outsiders: Studies in the Sociology of Deviance.* New York: Free Press.

Beckett, Katherine. 1996. "Culture and the Politics of Signification: The Case of Child Sexual Abuse." *Social Problems* 43(1): 57–76.

Bell, Ann V. 2014. *Misconception: Social Class and Infertility in America.* New Brunswick: Rutgers University Press.

Bell, Susan E. 2009. *DES Daughters: Embodied Knowledge and the Transformation of Women's Health Politics.* Philadelphia: Temple University Press.

Bell, Susan E. and Anne E. Figert, eds. 2015. *Reimagining (Bio)Medicalization, Pharmaceuticals, and Genetics: Old Critiques and New Engagements.* New York: Routledge.

Bello, Jennifer K., Goutham Rao, and Debra B. Stulberg. 2015. "Trends in Contraceptive and Preconception Care in United States Ambulatory Practices." *Family Medicine* 47(4): 264–71.

Bennet, John Cook. 1829. "An Account of a Singular Case of Fetal Monstrosity." *Boston Medical and Surgical Journal* 2: 650–51.

Berend, Zsuzsa. 2012. "The Romance of Surrogacy." *Sociological Forum* 27: 913–36.

Best, Joel. 1987. "Rhetoric in Claims-Making: Constructing the Missing Children Problem." *Social Problems* 34(2): 101–21.

Bish, Connie L., Sherry Farr, Dick Johnson, and Ron McAnally. 2012. "Preconception Health of Reproductive Aged Women of the Mississippi River Delta." *Maternal and Child Health Journal* 16 (Supp. 2): 250–57.

Bliss, Catherine. 2012. *Decoding Race: The Genomic Fight for Social Justice.* Stanford: Stanford University Press.

Blum, Linda. 1999. *At the Breast: Ideologies of Breastfeeding and Motherhood in the Contemporary United States.* Boston: Beacon Press.

BMJ. 1904. "Review: Antenatal Pathology." *British Medical Journal* 2(2294): 1643–44.

———. 1934. "Results of Ante-Natal Care." *British Medical Journal* 2(3839): 220–21.

———. 1981. "Preconception Clinics." *British Medical Journal* 283: 685.

———. 1991. "Maternity Services." *British Medical Journal* 302: 1174.

Boonstra, Heather D., Rachel Benson Gold, Cory L. Richards, and Lawrence B. Finer. 2006. *Abortion in Women's Lives.* New York: Guttmacher Institute.

Bowker, Geoffrey C. and Susan Leigh Star. 1999. *Sorting Things Out: Classification and Its Consequences.* Cambridge: MIT Press.

Brandt, Allan. M. 1985. *No Magic Bullet: A Social History of Venereal Disease in the United States since 1880.* New York: Oxford University Press.

Brandt, Allan. M. and Martha Gardner. 2000. "Antagonism and Accommodation: Interpreting the Relationship between Public Health and Medicine in the United States during the 20th Century." *American Journal of Public Health* 90: 707–15.

Brandt, Allan M. and Paul Rozin. 1997. "Introduction." In *Morality and Health,* edited by A. M. Brandt and A. P. Rozin. New York: Routledge.

Bridges, Khiara. 2011. *Reproducing Race: An Ethnography of Pregnancy as a Site of Racialization.* Berkeley: University of California Press.

Brink, Susan. 2013. *The Fourth Trimester: Understanding, Protecting, and Nurturing an Infant through the First Three Months.* Berkeley: University of California Press.

Bronstein, Janet M. 2016. *Preterm Birth in the United States: A Sociocultural Approach.* Springer International Publishing.

Brown, Phil. 1995. "Naming and Framing: The Social Construction of Diagnosis and Illness." *Journal of Health and Social Behavior* 35: 34–52.

Brush, Lisa D. 1996. "Love, Toil, and Trouble: Motherhood and Feminist Politics." *Signs: Journal of Women in Culture and Society* 21(21): 429–54.

Bucher, Rue. 1962/1972. "Pathology: A Study of Social Movements within a Profession." In *Medical Men and Their Work,* edited by E. Freidson and J. Lorber. Chicago: Aldine-Atherton. Pp. 113–27.

Burtle, Adam and Stephen Bezruchka. 2016. "Population Health and Paid Parental Leave: What the United States Can Learn from Two Decades of Research." *Healthcare* 4(2): 30.

Callegari, Lisa S., Abigail R. A. Aiken, Christine Dehlendorf, Patty Cason, and Sonya Borrero. 2016. "Addressing Potential Pitfalls of Reproductive Life

Planning with Patient-Centered Counseling." *American Journal of Obstetrics & Gynecology* 216(2): 129–34.

Campbell, Nancy D. 1999. "Regulating 'Maternal Instinct': Governing Mentalities of Late Twentieth-Century U.S. Illicit Drug Policy." *Signs* 24: 895–923.

Campo-Engelstein, Lisa, Laura Beth Santacrose, Zubin Master, and Wendy M. Parker. 2016. "Bad Moms, Blameless Dads: The Portrayal of Maternal and Paternal Age and Preconception Harm in U.S. Newspapers." *AJOB Empirical Bioethics* 7(1): 56–63.

Cancian, Francesca M. 1986. "The Feminization of Love." *Signs* 11: 692–709.

Cartier, Lola, Carol L. Clow, Abby Lippman-Hand, Jean Morissette, and Charles R. Scriver. 1982. "Prevention of Mental Retardation in Offspring of Hyperphenylalaninemic Mothers." *American Journal of Public Health* 72(12): 1386–90.

"Case Showing the Importance of Early Manual Examination in Cases of Threatened Abortion." 1824. *New England Journal of Medicine and Surgery* 13: 121–24.

Casey, Frances E., Freya L. Sonenstein, Nan M. Astone, Joseph H. Pleck, Jacinda K. Dariotis, and Arik V. Marcell. 2016. "Family Planning and Preconception Health among Men in Their Mid-30s: Developing Indicators and Describing Need." *American Journal of Men's Health* 10(1): 59–67.

Casper, Monica J. 1998. *The Making of the Unborn Patient: A Social Anatomy of Fetal Surgery*. New Brunswick: Rutgers University Press.

Casper, Monica J. and Lisa Jean Moore. 2009. *Missing Bodies: The Politics of Visibility*. New York: New York University Press.

Castel, Robert. 1991. "From Dangerousness to Risk." In *The Foucault Effect: Studies in Governmentality*, edited by G. Burchell, C. Gordon, and P. Miller. London: Harvester/Wheatsheaf. Pp. 281–98.

Cefalo, Robert C. and Merry-K. Moos. 1988. *Preconceptional Health Promotion: A Practical Guide*. Rockville, MD: Aspen Publishers, Inc.

———. 1995. *Preconceptional Health Care: A Practical Guide* (2nd ed.). St. Louis: Mosby.

Centers for Disease Control and Prevention (CDC). 1992. "Recommendations for the Use of Folic Acid to Reduce the Number of Cases of Spina Bifida and Other Neural Tube Defects." *Morbidity and Mortality Weekly Report* 41(RR-14): 001.

———. 2008 (January 11). "Update on Overall Prevalence of Major Birth Defects—Atlanta, Georgia, 1978–2005." *Morbidity and Mortality Weekly Report* 57(01): 1–5.

———. 2015 (October 9). "CDC Grand Rounds: Understanding the Causes of Major Birth Defects—Steps to Prevention." *Morbidity and Mortality Weekly Report* 64(39): 1104–07.

Chamberlain, Geoffrey. 1980. "The Prepregnancy Clinic." *British Medical Journal* 281(6232): 29–30.

Chang, Hannah H., Jim Larson, Hannah Blencowe, Catherine Y. Spong, Christopher P. Howson, Sarah Cairns-Smith, Eve M. Lackritz, Shoo K. Lee, Elizabeth Mason, Andrew C. Serazin, Salimah Walani, Joe Leigh Simpson, Joy E. Lawn, on behalf of the Born Too Soon Preterm Prevention Analysis Group. 2013. "Preventing Preterm Births: Analysis of Trends and Potential Reductions with Interventions in 39 Countries with Very High Human Development Index." *Lancet* 381(9862): 223–34.

Channing, Walter Jr. 1825. "On a Species of Premature Labor." *New England Journal of Medicine and Surgery* 14: 151–56.

Charmaz, Kathy. 2006. *Constructing Grounded Theory: A Practical Guide through Qualitative Analysis*. London: Sage Publications.

Choiriyyah, Ifta, Freya L. Sonenstein, Nan M. Astone, Joseph H. Pleck, Jacinda K. Dariotis, and Arik V. Marcell. 2015. "Men Aged 15–44 in Need of Preconception Care." *Maternal and Child Health Journal* 19(11): 2358–65.

Chuang, Cynthia H., Diana L. Velott, Carol S. Weisman, Christopher N. Sciamanna, Richard S. Legro, Vernon M. Chinchilli, Merry-K. Moos, Erica B. Francis, Lindsay N. Confer, Erik B. Lehman, and Christopher J. Armitage. 2015. "Reducing Unintended Pregnancies through Web-Based Reproductive Life Planning and Contraceptive Action Planning among Privately Insured Women: Study Protocol for the MyNewOptions Randomized, Controlled Trial." *Women's Health Issues* 25(6): 641–48.

Clarke, Adele E. 1998. *Disciplining Reproduction: Modernity, American Life Sciences, and the Problems of Sex*. Berkeley: University of California Press.

———. 2005. *Situational Analysis: Grounded Theory after the Postmodern Turn*. Thousand Oaks: SAGE.

Clarke, Adele E., Janet K. Shim, Laura Mamo, Jennifer Ruth Fosket, and Jennifer R. Fishman. 2003. "Biomedicalization: Technoscientific Transformations of Health, Illness, and U.S. Biomedicine." *American Sociological Review* 68(2): 161–94.

Clarke, Adele E., Laura Mamo, Jennifer Ruth Fosket, Jennifer R. Fishman, and Janet K. Shim, eds. 2010. *Biomedicalization: Technoscience, Health, and Illness in the U.S.* Durham: Duke University Press.

Clarke, Adele E. and Susan Leigh Star. 2007. "The Social Worlds Framework: A Theory/Methods Package." In *The Handbook of Science and Technology Studies* (3rd ed.), edited by E.J. Hackett, O. Amsterdamska, M. Lynch, and J. Wajcman. Cambridge: The MIT Press.

Clarke, Alison J. 2004. "Maternity and Materiality." *In Consuming Motherhood*, edited by J.S. Taylor, L.L. Layne, and D.F. Wozniak. New Brunswick: Rutgers University Press. Pp. 55–71.

Clarke, Edward H. 1873. *Sex in Education; Or, a Fair Chance for the Girls*. Boston: J.R. Osgood & Company.

Coale, Ansley J. 1973. "The Demographic Transition Reconsidered." In International Population Conference, Liege, Vol. 1. *Liege: International Union for the Scientific Study of Population*. Pp. 53–72.

Colen, Shellee. 1995. "'Like a Mother to Them': Stratified Reproduction and West Indian Childcare Workers and Employers in New York." In *Conceiving the New World Order: The Global Politics of Reproduction*, edited by F. D. Ginsburg and R. Rapp. Berkeley: University of California Press. Pp. 78–102.

Collins, H. M. 1985. *Changing Order: Replication and Induction in Scientific Practice*. London: SAGE Publications.

Collins, Patricia Hill. 2005. *Black Sexual Politics: African Americans, Gender, and the New Racism*. New York: Routledge.

Conrad, Peter. 1994. "Wellness as Virtue: Morality and the Pursuit of Health." *Culture, Medicine and Psychiatry* 18: 385–401.

———. 2007. *The Medicalization of Society: On the Transformation of Human Conditions into Treatable Disorders*. Baltimore: The Johns Hopkins University Press.

Conrad, Peter, and Miranda R. Waggoner. 2017. "Anticipatory Medicalization: Predisposition, Prediction, and the Expansion of Medicalized Conditions." In *Medical Ethics, Prediction, and Prognosis: Interdisciplinary Perspectives*, edited by M. Gadebusch-Bondio, F. Spöring, and J.-S. Gordon. London: Routledge. Pp. 95–103.

Conry, Jeanne A. 2013. "Presidential Address: Every Woman, Every Time." *Obstetrics & Gynecology* 122(1): 3–6.

Creager, Angela N. H. 2013. *Life Atomic: A History of Radioisotopes in Science and Medicine*. Chicago: The University of Chicago Press.

Cross, Raymond G. 1961. "Prevention of Anencephaly and Foetal Abnormalities by a Preconceptional Regimen." *Lancet* 278: 1124.

Cullum, Arlene S. 2003. "Changing Provider Practices to Enhance Preconceptional Wellness." *Journal of Obstetric, Gynecologic & Neonatal Nursing* 32(4): 543–49.

Cumston, Charles Greene. 1895. "Metritis as a Cause of Miscarriage." *Boston Medical and Surgical Journal* 133: 281–84.

Cunningham, F. Gary, Kenneth J. Leveno, Steven L. Bloom, Catherine Y. Spong, Jodi S. Dashe, Barbara L. Hoffman, Brian M. Casey, and Jeanne S. Sheffield, eds. 2014. *Williams Obstetrics* (24th ed.). McGraw-Hill Education.

Currie, Janet and Reed Walker. 2011. "Traffic Congestion and Infant Health: Evidence from E-Zpass." *American Economic Journal: Applied Economics* 3(1): 65–90.

Daniels, Cynthia R. 1993. *At Women's Expense: State Power and the Politics of Fetal Rights*. Cambridge: Harvard University Press.

———. 1997. "Between Fathers and Fetuses: The Social Construction of Male Reproduction and the Politics of Fetal Harm." *Signs* 22(3): 579–616.

———. 2006. *Exposing Men: The Science and Politics of Male Reproduction.* Oxford: Oxford University Press.

Darroch, Jacqueline E. 2006. "Family Planning: A Century of Change." In *Silent Victories: The History and Practice of Public Health in Twentieth Century America,* edited by J. W. Ward and C. Warren. New York: Oxford University Press.

Darroch, Jacqueline E., Susheela Singh, Jennifer J. Frost, and The Study Team. 2001. "Differences in Teenage Pregnancy Rates among Five Developed Countries: The Roles of Sexual Activity and Contraceptive Use." *Perspectives on Sexual and Reproductive Health* 33(6): 244–81.

Davis, Joseph E. 2016. "Reductionist Medicine and Its Cultural Authority." In *To Fix or to Heal: Patient Care, Public Health, and the Limits of Biomedicine,* edited by J. E. Davis and A. M. González. New York: New York University Press. Pp. 33–62.

Davis, Joseph E. and Ana Marta González. 2016. *To Fix or to Heal: Patient Care, Public Health, and the Limits of Biomedicine.* New York: New York University Press.

Department of Health and Human Services (DHHS). 1989. "Caring for Our Future: The Content of Prenatal Care. A Report of the Public Health Service Expert Panel on the Content of Prenatal Care." Washington, DC: Public Health Service, Department of Health and Human Services.

———. 2014. "The Health Consequences of Smoking: 50 Years of Progress. A Report of the Surgeon General." Atlanta, GA: U.S. Department of Health and Human Services, Centers for Disease Control and Prevention, National Center for Chronic Disease Prevention and Health Promotion, Office on Smoking and Health.

Dewees, William Potts. 1825. *A Treatise on the Physical and Medical Treatment of Children.* Philadelphia: Google Digital Books.

Douglas, Mary. 1992. *Risk and Blame: Essays in Cultural Theory.* London: Routledge.

Douglas, Mary and A. Wildavsky. 1982. *Risk and Culture: An Essay on the Selection of Technological and Environmental Dangers.* Berkeley: University of California Press.

Douglas, Susan J. and Meredith W. Michaels. 2004. *The Mommy Myth: The Idealization of Motherhood and How It Has Undermined Women.* New York: Free Press.

"Dropsy of the Amnion and Foetus." 1824. *New England Journal of Medicine and Surgery* 13: 360–66.

Dubos, René. 1959/1996. *Mirage of Health: Utopias, Progress, and Biological Change.* New Brunswick: Rutgers University Press.

Dubow, Sara. 2011. *Ourselves Unborn: A History of the Fetus in Modern America.* New York: Oxford University Press.

Duden, Barbara. 1993. *Disembodying Women: Perspectives on Pregnancy and the Unborn*. Cambridge: Harvard University Press.

Duggan, Lisa. 2003. *The Twilight of Equality?: Neoliberalism, Cultural Politics, and the Attack on Democracy*. Boston: Beacon Press.

Duster, Troy. 2003. *Backdoor to Eugenics*. New York: Routledge.

Einhorn, Amy. 2001. *The Fourth Trimester: And You Thought Labor Was Hard*. New York: Crown.

Epstein, Steven. 2007. *Inclusion: The Politics of Difference in Medical Research*. Chicago: The University of Chicago Press.

Faludi, Susan. 1991. *Backlash: The Undeclared War against American Women*. New York: Anchor Books.

Fennell, Julie Lynn. 2011. "Men Bring Condoms, Women Take Pills: Men's and Women's Roles in Contraceptive Decision Making." *Gender & Society* 25(4): 496–521.

Finer, Lawrence B. and Mia R. Zolna. 2011. "Unintended Pregnancy in the United States: Incidence and Disparities, 2006." *Contraception* 84: 478–85.

Finer, Lawrence B. and Stanley K. Henshaw. 2006. "Disparities in Rates of Unintended Pregnancy in the United States, 1994 and 2001." *Perspectives on Sexual and Reproductive Health* 38(2): 90–96.

Flavin, Jeanne. 2009. *Our Bodies, Our Crimes: The Policing of Women's Reproduction in America*. New York: New York University Press.

Fosket, Jennifer Ruth. 2010. "Breast Cancer Risk as Disease: Biomedicalizing Risk." In *Biomedicalization: Technoscience, Health, and Illness in the U.S.*, edited by A. E. Clarke, L. Mamo, J. R. Fosket, J. R. Fishman, and J. K. Shim. Durham: Duke University Press. Pp. 331–52.

Foucault, Michel. 1978/1990. *The History of Sexuality: Volume I*. Vintage Books.

———. 1988. "Technologies of the Self." In *Technologies of the Self: A Seminar with Michel Foucault*, edited by L. H. Martin, H. Gutman, and P. H. Hutton. Amherst: University of Massachusetts Press. Pp. 16–49.

Fournier, Barbara and George J. Fournier. 1980. *Pre-Parenting: A Guide to Planning Ahead*. Englewood Cliffs, NJ: Prentice Hall.

Franklin, Sarah and Celia Roberts. 2006. *Born and Made: An Ethnography of Preimplantation Genetic Diagnosis*. Princeton: Princeton University Press.

Fraser, Nancy. 1989. *Unruly Practices: Power, Discourse and Gender in Contemporary Social Theory*. Minneapolis: University of Minnesota Press.

Freda, Margaret Comerford and Ellen Tate Patterson. 1994. "Preterm Labor: Prevention and Nursing Management." *March of Dimes Nursing Modules*. White Plains, NY: March of Dimes Birth Defects Foundation.

Freda, Margaret Comerford, Merry-K. Moos, and Michele Curtis. 2006. "The History of Preconception Care: Evolving Guidelines and Standards." *Maternal and Child Health Journal* 10: 43–52.

Frey, Keith A., Shannon M. Navarro, Milton Kotelchuck, and Michael C. Lu. 2008. "The Clinical Content of Preconception Care: Preconception Care for Men." *American Journal of Obstetrics & Gynecology* 199: S389–95.

Frickel, Scott and Neil Gross. 2005. "A General Theory of Scientific/Intellectual Movements." *American Sociological Review* 70: 204–32.

Friedman, Emmeline, Megan S. Orlando, Jean Anderson, and Jenell S. Coleman. 2016. "'Everything I Needed from Her Was Everything She Gave Back to Me:' An Evaluation of Preconception Counseling for U.S. HIV-Serodiscordant Couples Desiring Pregnancy." *Women's Health Issues* 26(3): 351–56.

Friesen, Rhinehart F. 1970. "Pre-Pregnancy Care—a Logical Extension of Prenatal Care." *Canadian Medical Association Journal* 103(5): 495–07.

Gálvez, Alyshia. 2011. *Patient Citizens, Immigrant Mothers: Mexican Women, Public Prenatal Care, and the Birth-Weight Paradox.* New Brunswick: Rutgers University Press.

Gentile, Katie. 2013. "Biopolitics, Trauma and the Public Fetus: An Analysis of Preconception Care." *Subjectivity* 6(2): 153–72.

Geronimus, A. T. 2003. "Damned If You Do: Culture, Identity, Privilege, and Teenage Childbearing in the United States." *Social Science & Medicine* 57(5): 881–93.

Giddens, Anthony. 1991. *Modernity and Self-Identity: Self and Society in the Late Modern Age.* Stanford: Stanford University Press.

Gieryn, Thomas F. 1983. "Boundary-Work and the Demarcation of Science from Non-Science: Strains and Interests in Professional Ideologies of Scientists." *American Sociological Review* 48: 781–95.

———. 1999. *Cultural Boundaries of Science: Credibility on the Line.* Chicago: The University of Chicago Press.

Gilbert, G. Nigel and Michael Mulkay. 1984. *Opening Pandora's Box: A Sociological Analysis of Scientists' Discourse.* Cambridge: Cambridge University Press.

Gillespie, Chris. 2012. "The Experience of Risk as 'Measured Vulnerability': Health Screening and Lay Uses of Numerical Risk." *Sociology of Health & Illness* 24(2): 194–207.

Ginsburg, Faye D. and Rayna Rapp. 1995. "Introduction: Conceiving the New World Order." In *Conceiving the New World Order: The Global Politics of Reproduction*, edited by F. D. Ginsburg and R. Rapp. Berkeley: University of California Press. Pp. 1–17.

Glaser, Barney G. 1965. "The Constant Comparative Method of Qualitative Analysis." *Social Problems* (12): 436–45.

Glaser, Barney G. and Anselm L. Strauss. 1967. *The Discovery of Grounded Theory.* Chicago: Aldine.

Goethals, Thomas R. 1940. "Medical Aspects of Obstetrics." *New England Journal of Medicine* 222: 60–64.

Gold, Edwin M. 1955. "Perinatal Mortality." *Journal of the American Medical Association* 159: 244–47.

Gold, Rachel Benson. 2001. "Title X: Three Decades of Accomplishment." *The Guttmacher Report on Public Policy* 4(February): 5–8.

Goldstein, Bernard D. 2001. "The Precautionary Principle Also Applies to Public Health Actions." *American Journal of Public Health* 91: 1358–61.

Gordon, Linda. 1994. *Pitied but Not Entitled: Single Mothers and the History of Welfare*. New York: Free Press.

———. 2007. *The Moral Property of Women: A History of Birth Control Politics in America*. Urbana and Chicago: University of Illinois Press.

Grant, Adam M. and Amy Wrzesniewski. 2010. "I Won't Let You Down . . . Or Will I? Core Self-Evaluations, Other-Orientation, Anticipated Guilt and Gratitude, and Job Performance." *Journal of Applied Psychology* 95(1): 108–21.

Greene, Jeremy. 2007. *Prescribing by Numbers: Drugs and the Definition of Disease*. Baltimore: The Johns Hopkins University Press.

Greil, Arthur L. 1991. *Not Yet Pregnant: Infertile Couples in Contemporary America*. New Brunswick: Rutgers University Press.

Gurr, Barbara. 2015. *Reproductive Justice: The Politics of Health Care for Native American Women*. New Brunswick: Rutgers University Press.

Guttmacher Institute. 2016 (Sept.). "Fact Sheet: Contraceptive Use in the United States." http://www.guttmacher.org/pubs/fb_contr_use.html (accessed November 23, 2016).

Han, Sallie. 2013. *Pregnancy in Practice: Expectation and Experience in the Contemporary US*. New York: Berghahn Books.

Harvey, D. 2007. *A Brief History of Neoliberalism*. New York: Oxford University Press.

Hays, Sharon. 1996. *The Cultural Contradictions of Motherhood*. New Haven: Yale University Press.

Hellerstedt, Wendy L., Phyllis L. Pirie, Harry A. Lando, Susan J. Curry, Colleen M. McBride, Louis C. Grothaus, and Jennifer Clark Nelson. 1998. "Differences in Preconceptional and Prenatal Behaviors in Women with Intended and Unintended Pregnancies." *American Journal of Public Health* 88: 663–66.

Helme, T. Arthur. 1907. "An Address on the Unborn Child: Its Care and Its Rights. Delivered at the Annual Meeting of the Lancashire and Cheshire Branch, Manchester, June 20th, 1907." *British Medical Journal* 2(2434): 421–25.

Herman, Barry and Susan K. Perry. 1992/1997. *The Twelve-Month Pregnancy: What You Need to Know before You Conceive to Ensure a Healthy Beginning for You and Your Baby*. Los Angeles: Lowell House.

Heslin, J. A. and A. B. Natow. 1984. "Nutrition Needs for the Preconception Period." *Occupational Health Nursing* 32: 469–73.

Hewitt, H. P. 1939. "Preconceptional Care." *Southern Medical Journal* 32: 417–22.

Higgins, Jenny A., Jennifer S. Hirsch, and James Trussell. 2008. "Pleasure, Prophylaxis and Procreation: A Qualitative Analysis of Intermittent Contraceptive Use and Unintended Pregnancy." *Perspectives on Sexual and Reproductive Health* 40(3): 130–37.

Hilgartner, Stephen. 2000. *Science on Stage: Expert Advice as Public Drama.* Stanford: Stanford University Press.

Hilgartner, Stephen and Charles L. Bosk. 1988. "The Rise and Fall of Social Problems: A Public Arenas Model." *American Journal of Sociology* 94: 53–78.

Hird, Myra J. 2007. "The Corporeal Generosity of Maternity." *Body & Society* 13: 1–20.

Hollingsworth, Dorothy Reycroft, Oliver W. Jones, and Robert Resnik. 1984. "Expanded Care in Obstetrics for the 1980s: Preconception and Early Postconception Counseling." *American Journal of Obstetrics & Gynecology* 149: 811–14.

Honein, Margaret A., Leonard J. Paulozzi, T. J. Mathews, J. David Erickson, and Lee-Yang C. Wong. 2001. "Impact of Folic Acid Fortification of the US Food Supply on the Occurrence of Neural Tube Defects." *Journal of the American Medical Association* 285(23): 2981–86.

Hoppe, Trevor. 2013. "Controlling Sex in the Name of 'Public Health': Social Control and Michigan HIV Law." *Social Problems* 60(1): 27–49.

Horwitz, Allan V. and Jerome C. Wakefield. 2012. *The Loss of Sadness: How Psychiatry Transformed Normal Sorrow into Depressive Disorder.* New York: Oxford University Press.

Howell, Embry M. 2001. "The Impact of the Medicaid Expansions for Pregnant Women: A Synthesis of the Evidence." *Medical Care Research and Review* 58(1): 3–30.

Hutchins, Vince L. 1994. "Maternal and Child Health Bureau: Roots." *Pediatrics* 94(5): 695–99.

Ingamells, C. R. 1987. "Preconception Clinics (Letters)." *Journal of the Royal College of General Practitioners* 37(304): 510.

Institute of Medicine (IOM), Committee to Study the Prevention of Low Birthweight. 1985. *Preventing Low Birthweight: Summary.* Washington, DC: National Academy Press.

Jack, Brian. 1995. "Preconception Care (or How All Family Physicians Can 'Do' OB)." *American Family Physician* 51(8): 1807–08.

Jack, Brian W., Hani Atrash, Timothy Bickmore, and Kay Johnson. 2008. "The Future of Preconception Care: A Clinical Perspective." *Women's Health Issues* 18(6, Supp. 1): S19–S25.

Jack, Brian W. and Larry Culpepper. 1990. "Commentary: Preconception Care." *Journal of the American Medical Association* 264(9): 1147–49.

JAMA. 1932. "Proceedings of the New Orleans Session." *Journal of the American Medical Association* 98: 1889–1917.

———. 1940. "Tomorrow's Children: Proceedings of the First Southern Conference on Tomorrow's Children Held in Atlanta, Georgia, November 9–11, 1939." *Journal of the American Medical Association* 115: 638.

———. 1952. "The Chicago Session." *Journal of the American Medical Association* 148(15): 1281–339.

———. 1966. "Infant Mortality Key: Pre-Pregnancy Plans." *Journal of the American Medical Association* 197: 38–39.

Jasanoff, Sheila. 2004. *States of Knowledge: The Co-Production of Science and Social Order,* edited by S. Jasanoff. London: Routledge.

Jewell, David. 1990. "Preconception Clinics." *The Practitioner* 234(1486): 349–51.

Joffe, Carole. 2009. *Dispatches from the Abortion Wars: The Costs of Fanaticism to Doctors, Patients, and the Rest of Us.* Boston: Beacon Press.

Joffe, Carole and Jennifer Reich, eds. 2015. *Reproduction and Society: Interdisciplinary Readings.* New York: Routledge.

Johnson, Kay A. and Rebekah E. Gee. 2015. "Interpregnancy Care." *Seminars in Perinatology* 39: 310–15.

Johnson, Kay, Mary Balluff, Chad Abresch, Sarah Verbiest, and Hani Atrash. 2015. "Summary of Findings from the Reconvened Select Panel on Preconception Health and Health Care." Available at http://www.citymatch.org/sites/default/files/documents/002192_Preconception%20Health%20Report%20Booklet_5th.pdf (accessed Dec. 15, 2015).

Johnson, Kay, Samuel F. Posner, Janis Biermann, Jose F. Cordero, Hani K. Atrash, Christopher S. Parker, Sheree Boulet, and Michele G. Curtis. 2006. "Recommendations to Improve Preconception Health and Health Care—United States: A Report of the CDC/ATSDR Preconception Care Work Group and the Select Panel on Preconception Care." *Morbidity and Mortality Weekly Report* 55(RR06): 1–23.

Jones, Camara Phyllis, Benedict I. Truman, Laurie D. Elam-Evans, Camille A. Jones, Clara Y. Jones, Ruth Jiles, Susan F. Rumisha, and Geraldine S. Perry. 2013. "Using 'Socially Assigned Race' to Probe White Advantages in Health Status." In *Race, Ethnicity, and Health,* edited by T. A. LaVeist and L. A. Isaac. San Francisco: Jossey-Bass. Pp. 57–73.

Junod, Suzanne White. 2003. "Folic Acid Fortification: Fact and Folly." In *The Food and Drug Administration,* edited by M. A. Hickmann. New York: Nova Science Publishers, Inc. Pp. 55–62.

Kabat, Geoffrey C. 2008. *Hyping Health Risks: Environmental Hazards in Daily Life and the Science of Epidemiology.* New York: Columbia University Press.

Karp, Harvey. 2003. *The Happiest Baby on the Block.* Westminster, MD: Bantam.

Keely, Erin. 2012. "Preconception Care for Women with Type 1 and Type 2 Diabetes—the Same but Different." *Canadian Journal of Diabetes* 36: 83–86.

Kempner, Joanna. 2014. *Not Tonight: Migraine and the Politics of Gender and Health*. Chicago: The University of Chicago Press.

Klerman, Lorraine V. 1990. "A Public Health Perspective on 'Caring for Our Future'." *New Perspectives on Prenatal Care*, edited by I. R. Merkatz and J. E. Thompson. New York: Elsevier. Pp. 633–42.

———. 1997. "Promoting the Well-Being of Children: The Need to Broaden Our Vision—the 1996 Martha May Eliot Award Lecture." *Maternal and Child Health Journal* 1(1): 53–59.

———. 2006. "Family Planning Services: An Essential Component of Preconception Care." *Maternal and Child Health Journal* 10: 157–60.

Klerman, Lorraine V. and David W. Reynolds. 1994. "Interconception Care: A New Role for the Pediatrician." *Pediatrics* 93(2): 327–9.

Klerman, Lorraine V., Sharon L. Ramey, Robert L. Goldenberg, Sherry Marbury, Hou Jinrong, and Suzanne P. Cliver. 2001. "A Randomized Trial of Augmented Prenatal Care for Multiple-Risk, Medicaid-Eligible African American Women." *American Journal of Public Health* 91(1): 105–11.

Knight, Kelly Ray. 2015. *addicted.pregnant.poor*. Durham: Duke University Press.

Koven, Seth and Sonya Michel, eds. 1993. *Mothers of a New World: Maternalist Politics and the Origins of Welfare States*. New York: Routledge.

Krasner, Neville. 1984. "Alcohol Problems in Pregnancy and Childhood—Where Do We Go from Here?" *Alcohol & Alcoholism* 19(2): 181–84.

Krieger, Nancy. 1994. "Epidemiology and the Web of Causation: Has Anyone Seen the Spider?" *Social Science & Medicine* 39: 887–903.

Kukla, Rebecca. 2005. *Mass Hysteria: Medicine, Culture, and Mothers' Bodies*. Lanham, MD: Rowman & Littlefield Publishers, Inc.

———. 2010. "The Ethics and Cultural Politics of Reproductive Risk Warnings: A Case Study of California's Proposition 65." *Health, Risk & Society* 12(4): 323–34.

Ladd-Taylor, Molly and Lauri Umansky, eds. 1998. *"Bad" Mothers: The Politics of Blame in Twentieth-Century America*. New York: New York University Press.

Lamont, Michèle and Virág Molnár. 2002. "The Study of Boundaries in the Social Sciences." *Annual Review of Sociology* 28: 167–95.

Lancet. 1985. "Misconceptions About Preconceptional Care." *Lancet* 2: 1046–47.

Landsman, Gail H. 2009. *Reconstructing Motherhood and Disability in the Age of "Perfect" Babies*. New York: Routledge.

Lane, Christopher. 2007. *Shyness: How Normal Behavior Became a Sickness*. New Haven: Yale University Press.

Lappé, Martine. 2014. "Taking Care: Anticipation, Extraction and the Politics of Temporality in Autism Science." *BioSocieties* 9(3): 304–28.

———. 2016. "The Maternal Body as Environment in Autism Science." *Social Studies of Science* 46(5): 675–700.

Latour, Bruno. 1987. *Science in Action: How to Follow Scientists and Engineers through Society.* Cambridge: Harvard University Press.

Latour, Bruno and Steve Woolgar. 1979. *Laboratory Life: The Social Construction of Scientific Facts.* Princeton: Princeton University Press.

Laubenthal, Julian, Olga Zlobinskaya, Krzysztof Poterlowicz, Adolf Baumgartner, Michal R. Gdula, Eleni Fthenou, Maria Keramarou, Sarah J. Hepworth, Jos C. S. Kleinjans, Frederik-Jan van Schooten, Gunnar Brunborg, Roger W. Godschalk, Thomas E. Schmid, and Diana Anderson. 2012. "Cigarette Smoke–Induced Transgenerational Alterations in Genome Stability in Cord Blood of Human F1 Offspring." *FASEB Journal* 26(10): 3946–56.

Layne, Linda L. 2003. *Motherhood Lost: A Feminist Account of Pregnancy Loss in America.* New York: Routledge.

Lee, Ellie J. 2007. "Infant Feeding in Risk Society." *Health, Risk & Society* 9(3): 295–309.

Lesser, Arthur J. 1985. "Public Health Then and Now: The Origin and Development of Maternal and Child Health Programs in the United States." *American Journal of Public Health* 75(6): 590–98.

Lewis, Jan. 1997. "Mother's Love: The Construction of an Emotion in Nineteenth-Century America." *In Mothers & Motherhood: Readings in American History,* edited by R. D. Apple and J. Golden. Columbus: Ohio State University Press. Pp. 52–71.

Link, Bruce G. and Jo Phelan. 1995. "Social Conditions as Fundamental Causes of Disease." *Journal of Health & Social Behavior* 36(5):80–94.

Litt, Jacquelyn S. 2000. *Medicalized Motherhood: Perspectives from the Lives of African-American and Jewish Women.* New Brunswick: Rutgers University Press.

Lowe, Pam. 2016. *Reproductive Health and Maternal Sacrifice.* London: Palgrave Macmillan.

Lu, Michael C. 2009. *Get Ready to Get Pregnant: Your Complete Prepregnancy Guide to Making a Smart and Healthy Baby.* New York: Harper.

Lu, Michael C. and Kay A. Johnson. 2014. "Toward a National Strategy on Infant Mortality." *American Journal of Public Health* 104(S1): S13–S16.

Lu, Michael C., Keisher Highsmith, David de la Cruz, and Hani K. Atrash. 2015. "Putting the 'M' Back in the Maternal and Child Health Bureau: Reducing Maternal Mortality and Morbidity." *Maternal and Child Health Journal* 19(7): 1435–39.

Lu, Michael C., Milton Kotelchuck, Jennifer F. Culhane, Calvin J. Hobel, Lorraine V. Klerman, and John M. Thorp Jr. 2006. "Preconception Care between Pregnancies: The Content of Internatal Care." *Maternal and Child Health Journal* 10: 107–22.

Lu, Michael C. and Neal Halfon. 2003. "Racial and Ethnic Disparities in Birth Outcomes: A Life-Course Perspective." *Maternal and Child Health Journal* 7(1): 13–30.

Lu, Michael C., V. Tache, G. R. Alexander, M. Kotelchuck, and N. Halfon. 2003. "Preventing Low Birth Weight: Is Prenatal Care the Answer?" *Journal of Maternal-Fetal & Neonatal Medicine* 13(6): 362–80.

Luhmann, Niklas. 1993. *Risk: A Sociological Theory*. Translated by R. Barrett. New York: Aldine de Gruyter.

Luker, Kristin. 1985. *Abortion and the Politics of Motherhood*. Berkeley: University of California Press.

Luker, Kristin, Marjorie R. Sabel, Laurie Schwab Zabin, Christine A. Bachrach, Susan Newcomer, Linda S. Peterson, and William D. Mosher. 1999. "Forum: Contraceptive Failure and Unintended Pregnancy." *Family Planning Perspectives* 31(5): 248–53.

Lumley, Judith, P. S. Allen, Prue Plovanic, Carl Wood, and William Walters. 1980. "The Prepregnancy Clinic." *British Medical Journal* 281: 619.

Luna, Zakiya and Kristin Luker. 2013. "Reproductive Justice." *Annual Review of Law and Social Science* 9(1): 327–52.

Lupton, Deborah. 1995. *The Imperative of Health: Public Health and the Regulated Body*. London: SAGE.

———. 1999. "Risk and the Ontology of Pregnant Embodiment." In *Risk and Sociocultural Theory: New Directions and Perspectives*, edited by D. Lupton. Cambridge; New York: Cambridge University Press. Pp. 59–85.

———. 1999/2006. *Risk*. London: Routledge.

———. 2012. "'Precious Cargo': Foetal Subjects, Risk and Reproductive Citizenship." *Critical Public Health* 22(3): 329–40.

Lyerly, Anne Drapkin, Lisa M. Mitchell, Elizabeth Mitchell Armstrong, Lisa H. Harris, Rebecca Kukla, Miriam Kuppermann, and Margaret Olivia Little. 2009. "Risk and the Pregnant Body." *Hastings Center Report* 39(6): 34–42.

Lynch, M., L. Squiers, M. A. Lewis, R. Moultrie, J. Kish-Doto, V. Boudewyns, C. Bann, D. M. Levis, and E. W. Mitchell. 2014. "Understanding Women's Preconception Health Goals: Audience Segmentation Strategies for a Preconception Health Campaign." *Social Marketing Quarterly* 20(3): 148.

MacDorman, Marian F., Eugene Declercq, Howard Cabral, and Christine Morton. 2016. "Recent Increases in the U.S. Maternal Mortality Rate: Disentangling Trends from Measurement Issues." *Obstetrics & Gynecology* 128(3): 447–55.

MacDorman, Marian F. and T. J. Mathews. 2008. "Recent Trends in Infant Mortality in the United States." *NCHS Data Brief No. 9*. Hyattsville, MD: National Center for Health Statistics.

MacDorman, Marian F., T. J. Mathews, Ashna D. Mohangoo, and Jennifer Zeitlin. 2014. "International Comparisons of Infant Mortality and Related Factors: United States and Europe, 2010." *National Vital Statistics Reports* 63(5). Hyattsville, MD: National Center for Health Statistics.

MacKendrick, Norah A. 2014. "More Work for Mother: Chemical Body Burdens as a Maternal Responsibility." *Gender & Society* 28(5): 705–28.

MacKendrick, Norah and Lindsay S. Stevens. 2016. "'Taking Back a Little Bit of Control': Managing the Contaminated Body through Consumption." *Sociological Forum* 31(2): 310–29.

Malnory, Margaret E. and Teresa S. Johnson. 2011. "The Reproductive Life Plan as a Strategy to Decrease Poor Birth Outcomes." *Journal of Obstetric, Gynecologic & Neonatal Nursing* 40(1): 109–21.

Mamo, Laura, Amber Nelson, and Aleia Clark. 2010. "Producing and Protecting Risky Girlhoods." In *Three Shots at Prevention: The HPV Vaccine and the Politics of Medicine's Simple Solutions*, edited by K. Wailoo, J. Livingston, S. Epstein, and R. Aronowitz. Baltimore: The Johns Hopkins University Press. Pp. 121–45.

Mann, Emily S. 2013. "Regulating Latina Youth Sexualities through Community Health Centers: Discourses and Practices of Sexual Citizenship." *Gender & Society* 27(5): 681–703.

Mansfield, Becky. 2012a. "Gendered Biopolitics of Public Health: Regulation and Discipline in Seafood Consumption Advisories." *Environment and Planning D: Society and Space* 30(4): 588–602.

———. 2012b. "Race and the New Epigenetic Biopolitics of Environmental Health." *BioSocieties* 7(4): 352–72.

March of Dimes. 1993. "Toward Improving the Outcome of Pregnancy: The 90s and Beyond." White Plains, NY: March of Dimes Birth Defects Foundation.

———. 2002. "Is Early Prenatal Care Too Late? (March of Dimes Updates)." *Contemporary OB/GYN* 47(12): 54–72.

Marcus, George E. 1998. *Ethnography through Thick and Thin*. Princeton: Princeton University Press.

Markens, Susan. 1996. "The Problematic of Experience: A Political and Cultural Critique of PMS." *Gender & Society* 10(1): 42–58.

———. 2007. *Surrogate Motherhood and the Politics of Reproduction*. Berkeley: University of California Press.

———. 2012. "The Global Reproductive Health Market: U.S. Media Framings and Public Discourses about Transnational Surrogacy." *Social Science & Medicine* 74: 1745–53.

———. 2013. "'Is This Something You Want?': Genetic Counselors' Accounts of Their Role in Prenatal Decision Making." *Sociological Forum* 28(3): 431–51.

Markens, Susan, C. H. Browner, and Nancy Press. 1997. "Feeding the Fetus: On Interrogating the Notion of Maternal-Fetal Conflict." *Feminist Studies* 23(2): 351–72.

Martin, Emily. 1987/2001. *The Woman in the Body: A Cultural Analysis of Reproduction.* Boston: Beacon Press.

Martin, Lauren Jade. 2010. "Anticipating Infertility: Egg Freezing, Genetic Preservation, and Risk." *Gender & Society* 24(4): 526–45.

Massi, Lisa L. 2005. "Anticipated Guilt as Behavioral Motivation: An Examination of Appeals to Help Unknown Others through Bone Marrow Donation." *Human Communication Research* 31(4): 453–81.

Mathews, T. J. and B. E. Hamilton. 2002. "Mean Age of Mother, 1970–2000." *National Vital Statistics Reports* 51. Hyattsville, MD: National Center for Health Statistics.

Mathews, T. J., M. F. MacDorman, and M. E. Thoma. 2015. "Infant Mortality Statistics from the 2013 Period Linked Birth/Infant Death Data Set." *National Vital Statistics Reports* 65(9). Hyattsville, MD: National Center for Health Statistics.

McLanahan, Sara and Christine Percheski. 2008. "Family Structure and the Reproduction of Inequalities." *Annual Review of Sociology* 34: 257–76.

Meckel, Richard A. 1990. *Save the Babies: American Public Health Reform and the Prevention of Infant Mortality 1850–1929.* Baltimore: The Johns Hopkins University Press.

Meloni, Maurizio. 2016. *Political Biology: Science and Social Values in Human Heredity from Eugenics to Epigenetics.* New York: Palgrave Macmillan.

Metzl, Jonathan M. and Anna Kirkland, eds. 2010. *Against Health: How Health Became the New Morality.* New York: New York University Press.

Mills, James L., George G. Rhoads, Joe Leigh Simpson, George C. Cunningham, Mary R. Conley, Melinda R. Lassman, Margaret E. Walden, O. Richard Depp, and Howard J. Hoffman. 1989. "The Absence of a Relation between the Periconceptional Use of Vitamins and Neural-Tube Defects." *New England Journal of Medicine* 321(7): 430–35.

Minino, Arialdi M., Melonie P. Heron, Sherry L. Murphy, and Kenneth D. Kochanek. 2007. "Deaths: Final Data for 2004." *National Vital Statistics Reports* 55. Hyattsville, MD: National Center for Health Statistics.

Minkoff, Howard and Lynn M. Paltrow. 2006. "The Rights of 'Unborn Children' and the Value of Pregnant Women." *Hastings Center Report* 36(2): 26–28.

Misra, Dawn P., Bernard Guyer, and Adam Allston. 2003. "Integrated Perinatal Health Framework—a Multiple Determinants Model with a Life Span Approach." *American Journal of Preventive Medicine* 25(1): 65–75.

Misra, Dawn P. and Holly Grason. 2006. "Achieving Safe Motherhood: Applying a Life Course and Multiple Determinants Perinatal Health Framework in Public Health." *Women's Health Issues* 16(4): 159–75.

Mittal, Pooja, Aparna Dandekar, and Danielle Hessler. 2014. "Use of a Modified Reproductive Life Plan to Improve Awareness of Preconception Health in Women with Chronic Disease." *The Permanente Journal* 18(2): 28–32.

Monopoli, Mark L. 1995. "*McNulty v. McDowell*: Recognizing Preconception Tort in the Commonwealth?" *New England Law Review* 29: 763–94.

Montez, Jennifer Karas and Mark D. Hayward. 2011. "Early Life Conditions and Later Life Mortality." In *International Handbook of Adult Mortality*, edited by R. Rogers and E. Crimmins. Springer Publishers.

Moos, Merry-K. 2003. "Preconceptional Wellness as a Routine Objective for Women's Health Care: An Integrative Strategy." *Journal of Obstetric, Gynecologic & Neonatal Nursing* 32(4): 550–56.

———. 2006. "Preconception Health: Where to from Here?" *Women's Health Issues* 16(4): 156–58.

———. 2010. "From Concept to Practice: Reflections on the Preconception Health Agenda." *Journal of Women's Health* 19: 561–67.

Moos, Merry-K., Anne L. Dunlop, Brian W. Jack, Lauren Nelson, Dean V. Coonrod, Richard Long, Kim Boggess, and Paula M. Gardiner. 2008. "Healthier Women, Healthier Reproductive Outcomes: Recommendations for the Routine Care of All Women of Reproductive Age." *American Journal of Obstetrics & Gynecology* 199(6): S280–89.

Moos, Merry-K. and Robert. C. Cefalo. 1987. "Preconceptional Health Promotion: A Focus for Obstetric Care." *American Journal of Perinatology* 4(1): 63–67.

Moos, Merry-K., Shrikant I. Bangdiwala, Anne R. Meibohm, and Robert C. Cefalo. 1996. "The Impact of a Preconceptional Health Promotion Program on Intendedness of Pregnancy." *American Journal of Perinatology* 13(2): 103–08.

Morgan, Lynn. 2009. *Icons of Life: A Cultural History of Human Embryos*. Berkeley, CA: University of California Press.

Muller, F. and R. O'Rahilly. 1985. "The First Appearance of the Neural Tube and Optic Primordium in the Human Embryo at Stage 10." *Anatomy and Embryology* 172: 157–69.

Murkoff, Heidi and Sharon Mazel. 2009. *What to Expect before You're Expecting: The Complete Preconception Plan*. New York: Workman Publishing.

Nandi, Arijit, Mohammad Hajizadeh, Sam Harper, Alissa Koski, Erin C. Strumpf, Jody Heymann. 2016. "Increased Duration of Paid Maternity Leave Lowers Infant Mortality in Low- and Middle-Income Countries: A Quasi-Experimental Study." *PLOS Medicine* 13(3): e1001985.

National Center for Health Statistics (NCHS). 2001. "Healthy People 2000 Final Review." Hyattsville, MD: Public Health Service.

Nelson, Anita L., Salma Shabaik, Pamela Xandre, and Joseph Y. Awaida. 2016. "Reproductive Life Planning and Preconception Care 2015: Attitudes of

English-Speaking Family Planning Patients." *Journal of Women's Health* 25(8): 832–39.

Nettleton, Sarah. 1996. "Women and the New Paradigm of Health and Medicine." *Critical Social Policy* 16: 33–53.

Oakley, Ann. 1984. *The Captured Womb: A History of the Medical Care of Pregnant Women*. Oxford: Blackwell.

Oaks, Laury. 2001. *Smoking and Pregnancy: The Politics of Fetal Protection*. New Brunswick: Rutgers University Press.

Ogle, Amy and Lisa Mazzullo. 2011. *Before Your Pregnancy: A 90-Day Guide for Couples on How to Prepare for a Healthy Conception*. New York: Ballantine Books.

Opray, N., R.M. Grivell, A.R. Deussen, and J.M. Dodd. 2014. "Directed Preconception Health Programs and Interventions for Improving Pregnancy Outcomes for Women Who Are Overweight or Obese." *Cochrane Database of Systematic Reviews* (7).

O'Rahilly, Ronan. 1979. "Early Human Development and the Chief Sources of Information on Staged Human Embryos." *European Journal of Obstetrics & Gynecology and Reproductive Biology* 9(4): 273–80.

O'Rahilly, Ronan and Ernest Gardner. 1971. "The Timing and Sequence of Events in the Development of the Human Nervous System during the Embryonic Period Proper." *Anatomy and Embryology* 134(1): 1–12.

Oza-Frank, Reena, Rashmi Kachoria, Sarah A. Keim, and Mark A. Klebanoff. 2015. "Provision of Specific Preconception Care Messages and Associated Maternal Health Behaviors before and during Pregnancy." *American Journal of Obstetrics & Gynecology* 212(372): 1–8.

Page, Richard. 1981. "Preconception Clinics (Correspondence)." *British Medical Journal* 283: 858.

Paltrow, Lynn M. 2013. "*Roe v. Wade* and the New Jane Crow: Reproductive Rights in the Age of Mass Incarceration." *American Journal of Public Health* 103: 17–21.

Paltrow, Lynn M. and Jeanne Flavin. 2013. "Arrests of and Forced Interventions on Pregnant Women in the United States, 1973–2005: Implications for Women's Legal Status and Public Health." *Journal of Health Politics, Policy and Law* 38(2): 299–343.

Paul, Annie Murphy. 2010. *Origins: How the Nine Months Before Birth Shape the Rest of Our Lives*. New York: Free Press.

Pearce, Neil. 1996. "Traditional Epidemiology, Modern Epidemiology, and Public Health." *American Journal of Public Health* 86: 678–83.

Petchesky, Rosalind Pollack. 1987. "Fetal Images: The Power of Visual Culture in the Politics of Reproduction." *Feminist Studies* 13(2): 263–92.

Petersen, Alan and Deborah Lupton. 1996. *The New Public Health: Health and Self in the Age of Risk*. London: Sage Publications.

Petronis, Arturas. 2010. "Epigenetics as a Unifying Principle in the Aetiology of Complex Traits and Diseases." *Nature* 465(7299): 721–27.

Post, Abner. 1889. "Some Considerations Concerning Syphilis and Marriage." *Boston Medical and Surgical Journal* 121: 600–02.

Pugh, Allison J. 2009. *Longing and Belonging: Parents, Children, and Consumer Culture.* Berkeley: University of California Press.

Quadagno, Jill. 2015. "The Transformation of Medicaid from Poor Law Legacy to Middle-Class Entitlement?" In *Medicare and Medicaid at 50: America's Entitlement Programs in the Age of Affordable Care*, edited by A. B. Cohen, D. C. Colby, K. A. Wailoo, and J. E. Zelizer. New York: Oxford University Press.

Rabinow, Paul and Nikolas Rose. 2006. "Biopower Today." *BioSocieties* 1: 195–217.

Ragoné, Heléna. 1999. "The Gift of Life: Surrogate Motherhood, Game Donation, and Constructions of Altruism." In *Transformative Motherhood: On Giving and Getting in a Consumer Culture*, edited by L. Layne. New York: New York University Press. Pp. 65–88.

Rapp, Rayna. 2000. *Testing Women, Testing the Fetus: The Social Impact of Amniocentesis in America.* New York: Routledge.

Reader, F. C. and J. G. Grudzinskas. 1985. "Preconception Care." *The Practitioner* 229: 699–701.

Reagan, Leslie J. 2010. *Dangerous Pregnancies: Mothers, Disabilities, and Abortion in Modern America.* Berkeley: University of California Press.

Reardon, Jenny. 2004. *Race to the Finish: Identity and Governance in an Age of Genomics.* Princeton: Princeton University Press.

Reich, Jennifer A. 2014. "Neoliberal Mothering and Vaccine Refusal: Imagined Gated Communities and the Privilege of Choice." *Gender & Society* 28(5): 679–704.

———. 2016. *Calling the Shots: Why Parents Reject Vaccines.* New York: New York University Press.

"Reports of Societies: American Gynecological Society." 1903. *Boston Medical and Surgical Journal* 149: 379–81.

"Reports of Societies: Congress of American Physicians and Surgeons." 1894. *Boston Medical and Surgical Journal* 130: 589–95.

"Reports of Societies: Fortieth Annual Meeting of the American Medical Association." 1889. *Boston Medical and Surgical Journal* 121: 37–47.

Richardson, Sarah S. 2015. "Maternal Bodies in the Postgenomic Order: Gender and the Explanatory Landscape of Epigenetics." In *Postgenomics: Perspectives on Biology after the Genome*, edited by S. S. Richardson and H. Stevens. Durham: Duke University Press. Pp. 210–31.

Richardson, Sarah S., Cynthia R. Daniels, Matthew W. Gillman, Janet Golden, Rebecca Kukla, Christopher Kuzawa, and Janet Rich-Edwards. 2014 (August 14). "Society: Don't Blame the Mothers." *Nature* 512: 131–32.

Robbins, Cheryl L., Lauren B. Zapata, Sherry L. Farr, Charlan D. Kroelinger, Brian Morrow, Indu Ahluwalia, Denise V. D'Angelo, Danielle Barradas, Shanna Cox, David Goodman, Letitia Williams, Violanda Grigorescu, and Wanda D. Barfield. 2014 (April 25). "Core State Preconception Health Indicators—Pregnancy Risk Assessment Monitoring System and Behavioral Risk Factor Surveillance System, 2009." *Morbidity and Mortality Weekly Report* 63(SS03): 1–62.

Roberts, Dorothy. 1997. *Killing the Black Body: Race, Reproduction, and the Meaning of Liberty.* New York: Vintage Books.

———. 2009. "Race, Gender, and Genetic Technologies: A New Reproductive Dystopia?" *Signs* 34(4): 783–804.

Robertson, Horace B., Jr. 1979. "Toward Rational Boundaries of Tort Liability for Injury to the Unborn: Prenatal Injuries, Preconception Injuries and Wrongful Life." *Duke Law Journal* 1978(6): 1401–57.

Robinson, Joan H. 2016. "Bringing the Pregnancy Test Home from the Hospital." *Social Studies of Science* 46(5): 649–74.

Rockhill, B., I. Kawachi, and G. A. Colditz. 2000. "Individual Risk Prediction and Population-Wide Disease Prevention." *Epidemiological Reviews* 22(1): 176–80.

Rose, Geoffrey. 1985. "Sick Individuals and Sick Populations." *International Journal of Epidemiology* 14(1): 32–38.

Rose, Nikolas. 2007. *The Politics of Life Itself: Biomedicine, Power, and Subjectivity in the Twenty-First Century.* Princeton: Princeton University Press.

Rosenbaum, Sara. 2008. "Women and Health Insurance: Implications for Financing Preconception Health." *Women's Health Issues* 18(6) (Supp. 1): S26–S35.

Rosenberg, Charles E. 1976/1997. *No Other Gods: On Science and American Social Thought.* Baltimore: The Johns Hopkins University Press.

———. 2007. "Banishing Risk: Or, the More Things Change, the More They Remain the Same." In *Our Present Complaint: American Medicine, Then and Now.* Baltimore: The Johns Hopkins University Press. Pp. 60–76.

———. 2009. "Managed Fear." *Lancet* 373: 802–03.

Rosenblatt, Roger. A. 1989. "The Perinatal Paradox: Doing More and Accomplishing Less." *Health Affairs* 8(3): 158–68.

Rosenfield, Allan and Deborah Maine. 1985. "Maternal Mortality—a Neglected Tragedy: Where Is the M in MCH?" *Lancet* 2: 83–85.

Ross, Loretta J. 2006. *Understanding Reproductive Justice.* Atlanta: SisterSong.

Roth, Rachel. 2000. *Making Women Pay: The Hidden Costs of Fetal Rights.* Ithaca: Cornell University Press.

Rothman, Barbara Katz. 1989. *Recreating Motherhood.* New Brunswick: Rutgers University Press.

———. 1993. *The Tentative Pregnancy: How Amniocentesis Changes the Experience of Motherhood*. W.W. Norton & Company.

Rothman, Sheila M. 1978. *Woman's Proper Place: A History of Changing Ideals and Practices, 1870 to the Present*. New York: Basic Books.

Russell, Keith P. 1962. "The Compleat Obstetrician." *Journal of the American Medical Association* 181: 1023–25.

Ruzek, Sheryl Burt and Julie Becker. 1999. "The Women's Health Movement in the United States: From Grass-Roots Activism to Professional Agendas." *Journal of the American Medical Women's Association* 54: 4–8.

Salganicoff, Alina and Jane An. 2008. "Making the Most of Medicaid: Promoting the Health of Women and Infants with Preconception Care." *Women's Health Issues* 18S: S41–S46.

Seller, Mary J. 1982. "Preconception Care and Neural Tube Defects." *Midwife Health Visitor & Community Nurse* 18: 470–74.

Shapin, Steven and Simon Schaffer. 1985. *Leviathan and the Air Pump: Hobbes, Boyle, and the Experimental Life*. Princeton: Princeton University Press.

Sher, Jonathan. 2016. "Prepared for Pregnancy? Preconception Health, Education and Care in Scotland." NHS Greater Glasgow & Clyde (Public Health).

Shostak, Sara. 2010. "Marking Populations and Persons at Risk: Molecular Epidemiology and Environmental Health." In *Biomedicalization: Technoscience, Health, and Illness in the U.S.*, edited by A. E. Clarke, L. Mamo, J. R. Fosket, J. R. Fishman, and J. K. Shim. Durham: Duke University Press. Pp. 242–62.

———. 2013. *Exposed Science: Genes, the Environment, and the Politics of Population Health*. Berkeley: University of California Press.

Shwartz, Samuel. 1962. "Prenatal Care, Prematurity, and Neonatal Mortality." *American Journal of Obstetrics & Gynecology* 83: 591–98.

Silber, Bonnie Baxt. 1992. "Preconception Negligence: Where Is the Zone of Danger?" *Journal of Juvenile Law* 13: 66–79.

Skocpol, Theda. 1992. *Protecting Soldiers and Mothers: The Political Origins of Social Policy in the United States*. Cambridge: Belknap Press.

Smail, S. A. 1981. "Dietary Supplements in Pregnancy." *Journal of the Royal College of General Practitioners*. 31: 707–11.

Smithells, R. W., S. Sheppard, and C. J. Schorah. 1976. "Vitamin Deficiencies and Neural Tube Defects." *Archives of Disease in Childhood* 51: 944–50.

Smithells, R. W., S. Sheppard, C. J. Schorah, M. J. Seller, N. C. Nevin, R. Harris, A. P. Read, and D. W. Fielding. 1980. "Possible Prevention of Neural Tube Defects by Periconceptional Vitamin Supplementation." *Lancet* 315: 339–40.

Smith-Rosenberg, Carroll and Charles E. Rosenberg. 1976/1997. "The Female Animal: Medical and Biological Views of Women." In *No Other Gods: On Science and American Social Thought*, by C. E. Rosenberg. Baltimore: The Johns Hopkins University Press. Pp. 54–70.

Solinger, Rickie. 1992/2000. *Wake up Little Susie: Single Pregnancy and Race before* Roe v. Wade. New York: Routledge.

———. 2007. *Pregnancy and Power: A Short History of Reproductive Politics in America*. New York: New York University Press.

Solinger, Rickie and Mie Nakachi, eds. 2016. *Reproductive States: Global Perspectives on the Invention and Implementation of Population Policy*. New York: Oxford University Press.

Speert, Harold. 1980. *Obstetrics and Gynecology in America: A History*. Baltimore: Waverly Press.

Speller, V. M. 1981. "Preconception Clinics (Correspondence)." *British Medical Journal* 283: 858–59.

Star, Susan Leigh. 1983. "Simplification in Scientific Work: An Example from Neuroscience Research." *Social Studies of Science* 13: 205–28.

———. 1985. "Scientific Work and Uncertainty." *Social Studies of Science* 15: 391–427.

Star, Susan Leigh and James R. Griesemer. 1989. "Institutional Ecology, 'Translations' and Boundary Objects: Amateurs and Professionals in Berkeley's Museum of Vertebrate Zoology, 1907–39." *Social Studies of Science* 19: 387–420.

Stebbins, G. S. 1887. "A Case of Pregnancy in a Uterus Bilocularis." *Boston Medical and Surgical Journal* 116: 444–46.

Steefel, David S. 1977. "Preconception Torts: Foreseeing the Unconceived." *University of Colorado Law Review* 48: 621–40.

Steel, Judith M., F. D. Johnstone, A. F. Smith, and L. J. P. Duncan. 1982. "Five Years' Experience of a 'Prepregnancy' Clinic for Insulin-Dependent Diabetics." *British Medical Journal* 285: 353–56.

Stern, Alexandra Minna. 2005. *Eugenic Nation: Faults and Frontiers of Better Breeding in Modern America*. Berkeley: University of California Press.

Stevens, Lindsay M. 2015. "Planning Parenthood: Health Care Providers' Perspectives on Pregnancy Intention, Readiness, and Family Planning." *Social Science & Medicine* 139: 44–52.

———. 2016. "Environmental Contaminants and Reproductive Bodies: Provider Perspectives on Risk, Gender, and Responsibility." *Journal of Health and Social Behavior* 57(4): 471–85.

Strong, Thomas H. 2000. *Expecting Trouble: What Expectant Parents Should Know about Prenatal Care in America*. New York: New York University Press.

Sussman, John R. and B. Blake Levitt. 1989. *Before You Conceive: The Complete Prepregnancy Guide*. New York: Bantam Books.

Swidler, Ann. 1986. "Culture in Action: Symbols and Strategies." *American Sociological Review* 51(2): 273–86.

Szasz, Andrew. 2007. *Shopping Our Way to Safety: How We Changed from Protecting the Environment to Protecting Ourselves.* Minneapolis: University of Minnesota Press.

Takeshita, J.Y., J.Y. Peng, and P.K. Liu. 1964. "A Study of the Effectiveness of the Prepregnancy Health Program in Taiwan." *Eugenics Quarterly* 11: 222–33.

Taussig, Fred J. 1937. "The Control of Abortion." *New England Journal of Medicine* 216: 109–14.

Taylor, Janelle S. 2008. *The Public Life of the Fetal Sonogram: Technology, Consumption, and the Politics of Reproduction.* New Brunswick: Rutgers University Press.

Thompson, Erika L., Coralia Vázquez-Otero, Cheryl A. Vamos, Stephanie L. Marhefka, Nolan S. Kline, Ellen M. Daley. 2017. "Rethinking Preconception Care: A Critical, Women's Health Perspective." *Maternal and Child Health Journal* 21(5): 1147–55.

Thompson, Joyce E., Linda V. Walsh, and Irwin R. Merkatz. 1990. "The History of Prenatal Care: Cultural, Social, and Medical Contexts." In *New Perspectives on Prenatal Care,* edited by I.R. Merkatz and J.E. Thompson. New York: Elsevier. Pp. 9–30.

Timmermans, Stefan and Mara Buchbinder. 2010. "Patients-in-Waiting: Living Between Sickness and Health in the Genomics Era." *Journal of Health and Social Behavior* 51: 408–23.

Tolich, Martin. 2004. "Internal Confidentiality: When Confidentiality Assurances Fail Relational Informants." *Qualitative Sociology* 27(1): 101–06.

Toombs, Percy W. 1923. "Parenthood and Race Culture." *The Journal of Heredity* 14: 33–38.

Trussell, James, Barbara Vaughan, and Joseph Stanford. 1999. "Are All Contraceptive Failures Unintended Pregnancies? Evidence from the 1995 National Survey of Family Growth." *Family Planning Perspectives* 31(5): 246–47.

Van der Zee, B., I.D. de Beaufort, E.A.P. Steegers, and S. Denktas. 2013. "Perceptions of Preconception Counselling among Women Planning a Pregnancy: A Qualitative Study." *Family Practice* 30(3): 341–46.

Van Dyck, Peter C. 2010. "Celebrating 75 Years of Title V (Maternal and Child Health) and Re-exploring our Roots." *Maternal and Child Health Journal* 14: 817–21.

Van Ness, A.W. 1955. "A Review of the Prepregnancy Treatment Clinic in Respect to Fetal Salvage." *New York State Journal of Medicine* 55(22): 3255–61.

Ventura, Stephanie J., Joyce C. Abma, William D. Mosher, and Stanley K. Henshaw. 2008. "Estimated Pregnancy Rates by Outcome for the United States, 1990–2004." *National Vital Statistics Reports* 56: 1–26. Hyattsville, MD: National Center for Health Statistics.

Verbiest, Sarah, Christina Kiko Malin, Mario Drummonds, and Milton Kotelchuck. 2016. "Catalyzing a Reproductive Health and Social Justice Movement." *Maternal and Child Health Journal* 20(4): 741–48.

Waggoner, Miranda R. 2013. "Motherhood Preconceived: The Emergence of the Preconception Health and Health Care Initiative." *Journal of Health Politics, Policy and Law* 38: 345–71.

Waggoner, Miranda R. and Tobias Uller. 2015. "Epigenetic Determinism in Science and Society." *New Genetics and Society* 34(2): 177–95.

Wailoo, Keith A. 2011. *How Cancer Crossed the Color Line.* New York: Oxford University Press.

Wald, Nicholas. 1993. "Folic Acid and the Prevention of Neural Tube Defects." *Annals of the New York Academy of Sciences* 678: 112–29.

Wald, Nicholas and MRC Vitamin Study Research Group. 1991. "Prevention of Neural Tube Defects: Results of the Medical Research Council Vitamin Study." *Lancet* 338: 131–37.

Wallace, Maeve, Emily Harville, Katherine Theall, Larry Webber, Wei Chen, and Gerald Berenson. 2013. "Preconception Biomarkers of Allostatic Load and Racial Disparities in Adverse Birth Outcomes: The Bogalusa Heart Study." *Paediatric Perinatal Epidemiology* 27(6): 587–97.

Weed, Douglas L. 2004. "Precaution, Prevention, and Public Health Ethics." *Journal of Medicine and Philosophy* 29(3): 313–32.

Weisman, Carol S. 1998. *Women's Health Care: Activist Traditions and Institutional Change.* Baltimore: The Johns Hopkins University Press.

Wertz, Dorothy C. 2001. "Preconception Sex Selection: A Question of Consequences." *American Journal of Bioethics* 1: 36–37.

Weston, Kath. 2002. *Gender in Real Time: Power and Transcience in a Visual Age.* New York: Routledge.

Whitworth, Melissa and Therese Dowswell. 2009. "Routine Pre-Pregnancy Health Promotion for Improving Pregnancy Outcomes." *Cochrane Database of Systematic Reviews* (4).

WHO. 2012. "Meeting to Develop a Global Consensus on Preconception Care to Reduce Maternal and Childhood Mortality and Morbidity." *World Health Organization Meeting Report* (Feb. 6–7, 2012). Geneva.

WHO, March of Dimes, Partnership for Maternal, Newborn & Child Health, and Save the Children. 2012. "Born Too Soon: The Global Action Report on Preterm Birth." Geneva: World Health Organization.

Wilcox, Lynne S. 2002. "Introductory Commentary: Pregnancy and Women's Lives in the Twenty-First Century: The United States Safe Motherhood Movement." *Maternal and Child Health Journal* 6(4): 215–19.

Williams, David R. and Michelle Sternthal. 2010. "Understanding Racial-Ethnic Disparities in Health: Sociological Contributions." *Journal of Health and Social Behavior* 51(S): S15–S27.

Williams, Joan C. 2012. *Reshaping the Work-Family Debate: Why Men and Class Matter.* Cambridge: Harvard University Press.

Williams, Norma. 1980. "The Prepregnancy Clinic." *British Medical Journal* 281: 747.

Wise, Paul H. 2008. "Transforming Preconceptional, Prenatal, and Interconceptional Care into a Comprehensive Commitment to Women's Health." *Women's Health Issues* 18(6S): S13–S18.

Wolf, Joan B. 2011. *Is Breast Best? Taking on the Breastfeeding Experts and the New High Stakes of Motherhood.* New York: New York University Press.

Worcester, J. A. 1900. "Breast Feeding." *Boston Medical and Surgical Journal* 143: 361–63.

Xaverius, Pamela K. and Joanne Salas. 2013. "Surveillance of Preconception Health Indicators in Behavioral Risk Factor Surveillance System: Emerging Trends in the 21st Century." *Journal of Women's Health Issues* 22(3): 203–09.

Xu, Jiaquan, Kenneth D. Kochanek, Sherry L. Murphy, and Betzaida Tejada-Vera. 2010 (May 20). "Deaths: Final Data for 2007." *National Vital Statistics Reports* 58: 1–136. Hyattsville, MD: National Center for Health Statistics.

Yuval-Davis, Nira. 1997. *Gender & Nation.* London: Sage Publications.

Zabriskie, L. 1929. *Nurses Handbook of Obstetrics.* Philadelphia: Lippincott.

Zelizer, Viviana A. 1985. *Pricing the Priceless Child: The Changing Social Value of Children.* Princeton: Princeton University Press.

Zetka, James R. 2008a. "The Making of the 'Women's Physician' in American Obstetrics and Gynecology: Re-Forging an Occupational Identity and a Division of Labor." *Journal of Health and Social Behavior* 49(3): 335–51.

———. 2008b. "Radical Logics and Their Carriers in Medicine: The Case of Psychopathology and American Obstetricians and Gynecologists." *Social Problems* 55(1): 95–116.

Zola, Irving Kenneth. 1972. "Medicine As an Institution of Social Control." *Sociological Review* 20(4): 487–504.

Zschoche, Sue. 1989. "Dr. Clarke Revisited: Science, True Womanhood, and Female Collegiate Education." *History of Education Quarterly* 29(4): 545–69.

Index

abortion: legalization of, 48; political contexts and, 28–29; pre-pregnancy care and rate of, 181, 209n30; and reproductive politics, 102–5, 213n50, 218n31; and reproductive silos in health care, 109–13, 111*fig*, 172–73

abortion, spontaneous, 206n140, 208n23; chronic conditions and, 15; and "every woman, every time" approach, 128; expanding blame for, 180–81; in nineteenth century beliefs and practices, 38–39; in twentieth century beliefs and practices, 45, 51, 58

AbouZahr, Carla, 102

Adair, Fred, 46, 47

Adams, Vincanne, 25

addiction, and pre-pregnancy health, 16, 194n60

Affordable Care Act, 97, 108, 169, 211n35

alcohol: and birth defects, 88; CDC recommendations on, 1, 184–87; expanding reproductive surveillance and, 55–57; men and, 142, 185; and optimizing reproduction, 81–83, 87; pre-pregnancy messaging and, 14–15

Al-Gailani, Salim, 52–53

Almeling, Rene, 22

American College of Obstetricians and Gynecologists (ACOG): on pre-conception care, 61–62, 169, 207n164

American Medical Association, and history of pre-pregnancy care, 47, 50, 107

anticipatory medicine: and future risk, 91–94; reproductive life plan and, 137; rise of, 25

anticipatory motherhood, 27, 29; and anticipatory medicine, 92–94; consumer culture and, 148; cultivating the maternal future through, 165–68; maternalism and, 123; and pre-maternal devotion, 156–60, 157*fig*; and social order, 176. *See also* Show Your Love campaign, CDC

Apple, Rima, 166

Armstrong, Elizabeth Mitchell, 11, 35, 183, 194n63, 205n117

Arney, William Ray, 51

Aronowitz, Robert, 92

Atrash, Hani: on the "every woman, every time" approach, 128, 142, 143; leadership in pre-conception care, 69–70, 88–89; as moral entrepreneur, 98–101; on the politics of women's health funding, 120; on prenatal care, 86; on reproductive silos and bridging boundaries, 113, 114–15